# Seeds of Sovereignty

# Seeds of Sovereignty

## Critical Public Health, Radical Sisterhood, and the Fight for Agricultural Justice

Andrew L. Carter

OXFORD
UNIVERSITY PRESS

OXFORD
UNIVERSITY PRESS

Oxford University Press is a department of the University of Oxford. It furthers the University's objective of excellence in research, scholarship, and education by publishing worldwide. Oxford is a registered trade mark of Oxford University Press in the UK and in certain other countries.

Published in the United States of America by Oxford University Press
198 Madison Avenue, New York, NY 10016, United States of America.



CIP data is on file at the Library of Congress.

ISBN 9780197789360

ISBN 9780197789353 (hbk.)

DOI: 10.1093/9780197789391.001.0001

Printed by Marquis Book Printing, Canada

The manufacturer's authorized representative in the EU for product safety is Oxford University Press España S.A. of Parque Empresarial San Fernando de Henares, Avenida de Castilla, 2 – 28830 Madrid (www.oup.es/en or product.safety@oup.com). OUP España S.A. also acts as importer into Spain of products made by the manufacturer.

MIX
Paper | Supporting responsible forestry
FSC® C103567

*Dedicated to the loving memory of Dru Ann Carter*

*(1957–2011)*

# CONTENTS

# LIST OF FIGURES

# ACKNOWLEDGMENTS

*SEEDS OF SOVEREIGNTY* IS A labor of love and passion project that has allowed me to thread together my broad spectrum of thoughts, arguments, and intellectual pursuits over the past decade into one cohesive outlet. The content in the pages that follow and the motivations and perspectives that inform them do not exist in isolation and have been honed and cultivated by a diverse collective of family, friends, colleagues, and community members who have encouraged me, shown love, challenged my perspectives, and believed in my potential—even when others, including myself, didn't. Far from a comprehensive list, I will try to acknowledge everyone who contributed creatively, emotionally, spiritually, and intellectually to this project.

First and foremost, the scope of this research would not be possible without the perspectives and lived stories of the chapter leaders, members, and associated communities of the National Women in Agriculture Association (NWIAA). In particular, I would like to acknowledge Tammy Gray-Steele, her uncle George Roberts, and others in her extended family for allowing me to document their story within the bigger narrative of ACB farming history; Diana Collingwood and her colleagues Tafari Tzaddi and Jamal Rogers at the Virgin Islands Department of Agriculture, for welcoming me with open arms to St. Croix and introducing me to the in-depth history of the Crucian food system; Emmanuel Opde, Olaitan Ariyo, Patience Kpeda, and the collective of women who represent NWIAA's African chapters—I continue to be inspired by your palpable passion for agriculture and women empowerment; and Noreen Whitehead, the fearless leader of the Georgia Women in Agriculture Association—you are a true force in every community that you touch.

The journey of this book from its inceptive ideas to the final product has been deeply shaped by the foundations of my intellectual home and academic community of critical health communication (CHC) scholars. For a good portion of my life, I have grappled with broader questions related to social justice, equity, and "alternative" perspectives outside of the mainstream in the context of health and wellness, though I lacked the language and theoretical grounding to clearly and effectively articulate my ideas. CHC has equipped me with an intellectual toolkit and creative canvas to explore and hone my thoughts over time. Several colleagues in the CHC community have contributed to my intellectual growth—and by proxy, the philosophical grounding of this project. I have tremendous appreciation for Mohan Dutta, whose pioneering work in the Culture-Centered Approach and fearless activism has strongly influenced my journey as an academic. Shaunak Sastry, who was one of the first senior scholars to support and believe in my work early on in my career, has been an important collaborator and thought partner. Other CHC colleagues I would like to thank include Satveer Kaur-Gill, Sean Upshaw, Patrick Dillon, Craig Stewart, and Heather Zoller. Your support, rather via deep dinner conversations at conferences, co-authoring papers together, or general guidance and mentorship, has been invaluable to my growth as a scholar and activist.

I would also like to acknowledge my broader academic community who have played a supportive role in helping me see this project to the finish line. To my graduate school day-ones: Adam Alexander, you have been in my corner since I first started developing my thoughts on this work over ten years ago, and Kalemba Kizito, your consistency as a friend, sounding board, and moral support made this project what it is. To my office mates, Vicky Gomez, who gave me the initial push I needed to begin writing this book after months of contemplation, and Rachel Berkowitz, who continuously lent an ear and moral support during our many hallway conversations when I was struggling to see this project's vision—I appreciate you having my back. I would also like to acknowledge my former and current colleagues at the University of Memphis' Department of Communication and Film and School of Public Health and San Jose State University's Department of Communication Studies, Department of Public Health and Recreation, and the Office of Diversity, Equity, and Inclusion. I am grateful for your collaboration and fellowship, whether you played an active role in supporting me through the writing process or were there during the earlier stages of my intellectual journey.

To my family: you were my primary motivation behind this manuscript—*Seeds of Sovereignty* is for you! Thank you, Dad and Lauren, for always being by my side. My motivation and interest in documenting a story about Black women farmers was cultivated by the many bold and pioneering Black women who helped raise me. To Grandma Mary, the matriarch who made this whole thing possible, I am continually grateful for your grace and wisdom (at your young age of 94). To my aunts, Sheri, Lisa, Denise, and Deb, thank you for being such strong examples in my life. Your friendship and trust mean the world to me. To my uncles, Reg, Pete, and Emmitt, your examples of healthy masculinity and love and support have shaped the person I am today. To my nieces Camberlynn and Kaia and nephew "Mr." Trent, thank you for bringing so much joy, laughter, and light into my life. You are next up—I am excited to see you take the mantle and run with it.

Lastly, to Dr. Nura Sediqe, I appreciate your partnership and continued fierce belief in me. The journey for this manuscript took us on writing retreats literally all over the world, from eclectic coffee shops in Brooklyn, San Francisco, Los Angeles, and Washington D.C., to picturesque backdrops in Tahiti, Sydney, and St. Thomas. Sharing the unique experience of writing our books side by side has been such a special journey. Thank you for your support, inspiration, and for making this chapter of life even more meaningful.

# I

# "Far, few, in between"

## Black Women Farmers, Foodways, and Critical Public Health Praxis

BLARING GUITAR RIFFS AND SAXOPHONE growls flow out of the endless row of bustling jazz clubs. The perpetual thrum and rustle of folks intermingling and cars whizzing by undergird the soundtrack of a vibrant business district packed with restaurants, hotels, and medical offices. An expansive cityscape reflects a plentitude of luxurious multistory homes, retail buildings, and large-scale development projects. More apt to epitomize the landscape of a contemporary metropolitan city, the Greenwood District in Tulsa, Oklahoma, emerged as a key cultural reference point and was exemplary of Black community sovereignty and self-reliance in the early twentieth century. Situated against the backdrop of historic forms of racial segregation and discrimination, the thriving neighborhood, eponymously known as "America's Black Wall Street," illuminated the potentialities for Black sustainability and economic transformation in the face of structural violence and inequity.

Black Wall Street largely came about as a result of the Land Run of 1889, where many freed Black Americans migrated to the Unassigned

*Seeds of Sovereignty*. Andrew L. Carter, Oxford University Press. © Oxford University Press (2026).
DOI: 10.1093/9780197789391.003.0001

Lands in Oklahoma following the forced removal of the Muscogee and Seminole peoples from their land via the Indian Removal Act of 1830. During the early 1900s, Black communities still faced the widespread impacts of Jim Crow segregation and were not allowed to make purchases or own businesses in predominantly white neighborhoods. Oklahoma, in particular, had some of the harshest and unjust Jim Crow laws in the United States (Small, 2020). Nonetheless, the region provided solace from Deep South segregation and the region's growing oil and mining industries made Tulsa an attractive option for many Black families and entrepreneurs, who fervently traveled by wagon, horse, train, and foot in hopes that a majority-Black population could foster community building and support economic and social mobilization. As the population grew and residents were forced, by circumstance, to buy from each other, capital quickly circulated throughout the Greenwood District community, engendering a fierce entrepreneurial spirit that birthed an expansive infrastructure of Black-owned businesses. At the height of Greenwood's vibrancy in 1921, the district encompassed 191 businesses owned by Black entrepreneurs (Messer et al., 2018).

Yet, despite the unbridled potential of Greenwood as a Black economic and political power center, its lifespan was short-lived. As Greenwood became more prosperous, it quickly multiplied, both in terms of population and geographic size. This widespread growth eventually spilled over into the boundaries of local white neighborhoods, leading many white residents to display resentment over the vast prosperity and rise of Black Wall Street. On May 31, 1921, the combustible climate burst into literal and figurative flames when, after the men of Greenwood (many of whom were former World War I veterans) assembled to protect a young Black man from getting lynched following accusations of attempted assault of a white woman on an elevator, a mob of angry white residents stormed the district in response, ultimately looting homes and businesses and burning them to the ground.[1] After the chaos ensued the following

[1] During the Jim Crow era, false or exaggerated allegations of sexual violence by Black men against white women were often weaponized to perpetuate the myth of Black men as inherently dangerous and hypersexual, a common trope steeped in white supremacist logics to justify de facto segregation and systemic oppression (Dray, 2007; Wells-Barnett, 1894).

day, thirty-six people were left dead, several thousand were left homeless, and more than thirty-five square blocks of Greenwood were decimated.

The Tulsa Race Massacre of 1921 is considered one of the worst incidents of racial violence in American history. While many historians and academics frame the incident as an isolated event, it is important to note that the legacy of Greenwood and Black Wall Street is intricately connected within a complex web of other Black economic sovereignty and political freedom movements throughout history that were surveilled and ultimately eradicated by white hegemonic power structures, such as the Memphis Massacre of 1866 in Memphis, Tennessee, the Wilmington insurrection of 1898 in Wilmington, North Carolina, the Springfield Race Riot of 1908 in Springfield, Illinois, the Rosewood Massacre of 1923 in Rosewood, Florida, and, more recently, the Black Panther Party Movement and its Free Food "Survival" Programs in Oakland, California during the 1960s. At the same time, the unique social circumstances and cultural context of the moment offer a blueprint toward the possibilities of Black self-reliance and economic sovereignty in the twenty-first century.

Today, there are no longer de jure segregation laws and many (overt) forms of racial discrimination in 1920s America are a faded memory. Nonetheless, new and more insidious forms of structural racism and inequity spawn continuously to inflict pervasive violence on Black communities—requiring the need for innovative strategies that make transparent and counteract such injustices. Today, located ninety minutes southwest of the Greenwood District in the heart of Oklahoma City, the evolution of a new Black Wall Street is quietly building force—this one led by a multigenerational collective of Black women using agriculture as their political weapon of choice to radically empower local and global communities and resist decades of erasure and violence. This book brings to light their story.

## Seeds of Sovereignty

"We are something that's national, that's never really been done before because on a local level, you see us unable to connect, because we're far, few, in-between. But powerhouses in each state, now internationally, we can share knowledge and we can bring our grant

dollars together once awarded, and massively impact our food chain. So, when this food system fails, we got something to fall back on."
— DARCEIA, *Texas chapter leader, National Women in Agriculture Association*

The above excerpt emerged out of a conversation I had during the National Women in Agriculture Association's (NWIAA) fifteenth anniversary conference on February 18, 2023. The three-day event, hosted at NWIAA's headquarters in Oklahoma City, Oklahoma, brought together leadership from the organization's national and international chapters in Africa, the Caribbean, and the United States to build capacity and strategize ways to engage policymakers around agricultural reform and food security issues. NWIAA was founded in 2008 by Tammy Gray-Steele, a former lawyer and fourth-generation farmer, who developed the organization as a way to address gendered inequities in agriculture and empower local Black farming communities across the United States. Starting with six original state chapters (i.e., Oklahoma, Georgia, Tennessee, Mississippi, Alabama, and Texas), NWIAA would add several chapters across the United States over the next decade. In 2020, with the realization that Black food security is intimately connected to broader disparities across global African, Caribbean, and Black (ACB)[2] communities, Tammy connected with several African women farmers while attending the Department of State's US-Africa Business Forum in Washington D.C., to develop a transnational connection with the addition of five NWIAA chapters in Nigeria. In 2021, NWIAA combined efforts with leadership at the Virgin Islands Department of Agriculture to develop a chapter in St. Croix, the United States Virgin Islands (USVI), strengthening this diasporic network across the Caribbean. In the years to follow, additional African chapters in Kenya, Liberia, Ghana, Malawi, Uganda, South Africa, and additional states in Nigeria would join the organization.

Today, NWIAA is considered one of the largest nonprofits for ACB women in agriculture globally, representing a diverse collective

---

[2] Black/African refers to persons with Sub-Saharan African ancestral origins with Brown or Black complexion. The term Black or African American signifies a geographical origin or African descent with attempts to describe a cultural group. Caribbean refers to the people, culture, and communities that are of African descent and reside in the Caribbean (Agyemang et al., 2005).

of multigenerational women across diverse contexts. The organization consists of seventy national chapters and nineteen international chapters spanning Africa and the Caribbean. Each chapter comprises various programs and support initiatives dedicated to serving a diverse array of stakeholders, including youth, young women, people with disabilities, and veterans.[3] As an asset-based, upstream public health model, NWIAA offers a fresh perspective for thinking about community food security across global ACB contexts.

The chapters that follow examine the lived stories, political strategies, social challenges, and locally situated knowledge of ACB women in agriculture to offer insight into how they support community food security, preserve cultural heritage, and restore frayed transnational cultural foodways. I make several claims throughout the book. Centrally, I argue that public health conversations on food security disparities must first explore how upstream inequities (e.g., land inaccessibility and ownership, food production disparities, agricultural policies) impact downstream consumption and access issues (e.g., food deserts, diet-related health disparities), rather than solely focusing resources and interventions on the latter (e.g., education/awareness campaigns, charity programs). Top-down agricultural and public health leaders can learn a lot from ACB women farmers' philosophical approach to growing and distributing food; to this point, I argue that their historical legacies, political identity, and shared deep-rooted agricultural knowledge offer an innovative and emancipatory model for rethinking asset-based, upstream public health interventions, particularly those focused on low-income communities and communities of color. Drawing on a combination of ethnographic and participatory action research, critical analyses, and observations, this book highlights the capacity of community-based and led, multi-sector (e.g., grassroots and grasstops)

[3] For example, some of the primary programs at the NWIAA headquarters location in Oklahoma City, Oklahoma include Bumblebee's and Butterflies (a farm education program where youth ages 6–12 learn to grow their own food), Junior Agri-Diva Education (J.A.D.E.), (a small business incubator program for young women ages 12 and up), Circle "R" Ranch (a program dedicated to helping young children with disabilities by integrating therapeutic activities with exposure to farm animals and nature), Free Fresh Produce Program (a community garden that provides free produce and harvesting education to local North Oklahoma residents), and Soil Sisters (a gardening program for women 65+).

political organizing and advocacy strategies to preserve cultural foodways and promote food security. At the same time, it documents the structural limitations and emancipatory potential of such approaches as they situate within existing social relations fraught with broader racial, patriarchal, political, cultural, and economic constraints.

At the heart of *Seeds of Sovereignty* is a story about food, health, and the unrelenting fight for community and global justice. The research for this book emerged amid the backdrop of multiple intersecting social crises. In 2020, the twin exigencies of the COVID-19 pandemic and the murder of George Floyd sparked global protests and uncovered marked disparities in health outcomes and access to resources among marginalized communities—mapping neatly along what Ruha Benjamin (2020) describes as "well-worn patterns of inequity." Paralleling these crises is the relentless and escalating threat of climate change, which poses severe social, environmental, and public health risks disproportionately impacting low-income communities and communities of color. These combined challenges have forced global society to critically interrogate the social structures that organize collective life and how they reproduce inequitable outcomes.

In the context of food security and access, the current structuring of the industrialized food system has resulted in multi-pronged crises that reproduce injustices across health, built environment, and social contexts (Borras & Mohamed, 2020; Neff et al., 2009; Passidomo, 2013; Gordon et al., 2022). During the height of the pandemic, snapshots of desolate grocery store shelves, closed food processing plants, milk vats being dumped, and pounds of expired eggs being smashed emerged from around the world, highlighting the precariousness of our food chain from farm to disposal. At the level of food production, the collective crises revealed marked inequities in *who* gets to be and be remembered as[4] a farmer, own land, receive support, and has capacity to

[4] Alison Alkon and Christine McCullen (2011) have explored the social and political influences embedded in who gets *to be remembered* as a farmer in their concept of the "white farm imaginary," which frames the small-scale, yeoman farmer as the quintessential American agricultural icon. This romanticized construct centers white farmer and landowner experiences in dominant agriculture narratives, while erasing the vital contributions of Black farmers and other farmers of color, whose labor is equally if not more essential to sustaining American agriculture.

remain resilient in the face of environmental and social catastrophe. For global ACB farming communities, these inequities are situated within a deep historical struggle of subjugation and cultural and knowledge co-optation.

## "Far, Few, in Between"

In the United States, the influence of Black farmers is built into the very foundations of modern agriculture and the food system, yet their contributions are erased from mainstream food and farming conversations. Black farmers were initially brought over in the Transatlantic slave trade by white landowners who did not possess their unique agrarian ingenuity and cultural knowledge (Littlefield, 1991). During the renaissance of Black farming in the 1920s, Black farmers represented 14 percent of the US farming population (926,000), while the overall Black population comprised only 10 percent of the national populace, demonstrating that the country had the capacity to support equitable conditions in agriculture (Penniman, 2018). However, since that time, Black farmers have lost land at a rate of almost 50 percent every decade, nearly tripling the loss of land of white farmers during the same period (Grant et al., 2012; Wood & Gilbert, 2000). Several factors have contributed to this decline, including discriminatory policies, institutionalized racism, the mechanization of agriculture and increases in agricultural technology, communicative and cultural erasure and co-optation, among others (Daniel, 2013; Hinson & Robinson, 2008). These collective influences have engendered the current uneven landscape in agricultural production and access to food and resources among Black communities.

Today, Black farmers in the United States are a dwindling and nearly extinct population, as they account for only 1.4 percent of the nation's farmers (48,697 producers), represent just 0.5 percent of farmland ownership (4.7 million acres), and 0.4 percent of total agriculture sales ($1.4 billion; USDANASS, 2017a). In an era of intersecting social crises, Black farmers are particularly vulnerable to the impacts of climate change, which threaten to further marginalize their existence and influence. For example, they have disproportionately fewer financial resources to invest in new technologies and infrastructure to mitigate climate risks in comparison to their white counterparts, and low political power to advocate for policies that support climate resilience (Akamani, 2021). Moreover, Black-owned farms are smaller in comparison to white-owned farms,[5] making them less adaptable to severe weather events, such as droughts, floods, hurricanes, and other extreme events exacerbated by climate change. Black farmers are also disproportionally impacted by environmental injustices caused by climate change; they are more likely to live and work in areas with poor air quality, contaminated water sources, and other environmental hazards (Bikomeye et al., 2021).

For Black women farmers, this uphill battle is even more arduous. Black women farmers face unique intersectional barriers to participation in the modern agricultural landscape, such as race, gender, class, and cultural marginalization, creating a cumulative effect that upholds disparities in access to climate change resources, community health outcomes, land ownership, and social capital (Leslie et al., 2019; Tyler & Fraser, 2016). Today, despite record numbers of female farmers entering the agricultural industry over the past decade, most are white (95 percent; 1.1 percent Black, respectively; USDANASS, 2017b) and non-operating landowners (513,000 White, 22,000 People-of-Color, respectively; Horst & Marion, 2019); this "1% of the 1%" reality is reflective of marked disparities in access to inherited land and wealth and credit to purchase land (Horst & Marion, 2019).

Historically, Black women have played an integral role in upholding the cultural and social fabric of their communities—be it through social movements, intellectual leadership, community health, or preserving art and culture—they remain irreplaceable in the interminable struggle for Black freedom. Whenever Black women are not centrally featured in leadership roles, their diminished existence often serves as a "canary in the coalmine," signaling deeper issues about the collective strength

[5] 85 percent of Black-owned farms had fewer than 180 acres (average size of 132 acres) and 57 percent had sales and government payments of less than $5,000/year in comparison to 431 acres and 47 percent white-owned operations, respectively (USDANASS, 2017a).

and well-being of their communities. In agricultural contexts, the eradication of Black women farmers represents more than a mere census data footnote or chalking up of "the way things are" in today's landscape but symbolizes the erasure of a rich legacy responsible for upholding many Black sovereignty and community food security movements throughout history and linking together shared diasporic political legacies and cultural foodways.

## ACB Cultural Foodways and Women Farmers Legacy

Foodways are understood as the cultural, social, and economic practices related to the production, distribution, preparation, and consumption of food within a particular community or society; they encompass everything from agricultural techniques and culinary traditions to food rituals and beliefs surrounding food, and often reflect a region's history, geography, climate, and cultural diversity, and shape how communities interact with and perceive food (Wright et al., 2021). In response to the myriad environmental, public health, and economic risks of the global food system, emerging research has explored the role of foodways as an entry point for addressing social inequities and developing multi-sector solutions (Cachelin et al., 2019; Cannuscio et al., 2010). Interdisciplinary researchers in fields such as critical food studies, environmental sustainability, and communication have theorized new ways to leverage foodways as a guiding framework for health and food justice praxis (Forson & Counihan, 2013; Leeds-Hurwitz, 2016). Though promising, much of this work is focused on the down and midstream components of the food system, such as how local communities navigate and make sense of their local food environments and develop shared meaning and identity around food. There is limited discussion on how food producers and broader production processes influence local foodways. In farming and agriculture, the erasure of Black women farmers has fractured ACB transnational foodways by disrupting collective memory and cultural knowledge.

For ACB communities, past and present structures of settler colonialism, racial and gendered capitalism, and structural violence have split up these once-linked foodways (Lunsford et al., 2021). Before the early 1500s, before colonization processes took shape, African foodways were diverse and varied, reflective of the continent's vast geography and cultural diversity. They were situated within a tropical coastal climate where people lived by hunting, fishing, foraging, cultivating wild foods, domesticating animals, and growing gardens and crops based on local ecosystems and cultures. The transatlantic slave trade in the 1600s involved the forced kidnapping, transportation, and enslavement of over 12 million indigenous Africans by European colonial powers to different regions across the world, including the Caribbean and the Americas. Slavery disrupted traditional African agricultural practices, dietary habits, and culinary traditions in myriad ways, leading to the fragmentation and loss of traditional African food systems. Following the abolition of slavery in the latter part of the nineteenth century, the African diaspora spanned diverse global regions. ACB foodways incorporated a combination of preserved agricultural practices and culinary traditions with influences from geographic-specific locations.

In the Caribbean, foodways reflected a mixture of African traditions with European, Spanish, and Indigenous Caribbean culinary practices. In the United States, despite deep-seated forms of structural violence, Black Americans preserved elements of their culinary heritage by drawing on centuries of agricultural knowledge and skill (e.g., crop cultivation, foraging, and hunting) and adapting traditional "soul food" culinary traditions to their constrained food availability and cooking methods in the US South. In West Africa, further forms of colonization resulted in the fragmentation and disruptions in traditional agricultural practices and food systems, such as land dispossession, cash crop production, and the introduction of Western crops and livestock.

The early to mid-twentieth century witnessed another transformation of ACB foodways as a result of white supremacy and racial capitalism. In the United States, a combination of Jim Crow segregation laws, co-optation and erasure of African food culture, and prevalent inequities in the dominant food system (e.g., food access and insecurity disparities, Black farming erasure) further divorced Black Americans from traditional African foodways (Cooley, 2015). In Caribbean contexts, the enduring impact of European colonization had lasting implications on Caribbean culinary traditions and agriculture. For example, European settlers introduced new crops, farming techniques, and livestock to the region, significantly transforming local agricultural practices. Further, the colonial plantation system prioritized the cultivation of cash "commodity" crops, which replaced the production of traditional fruit and vegetable crops—largely mirroring trends to come in the following decades by dominant global agribusiness models. Similarly, in West Africa, a combination of globalization and increased promotion of agricultural biotechnology largely erased many traditional agricultural practices and forced reliance on new seed and crop variations (O'Grady-Walsh, 2019).

Despite these long-standing forms of oppression and cultural violence, ACB women have fought valiantly throughout history to preserve cultural foodways, farming and cooking techniques, and indigenous knowledge among diasporic communities. Dating back to slavery, evidence suggests that many African women braided seeds into their hair as a means for survival of themselves and the cultural traditions of their homeland during the middle passage (Tyler, 2020). In Caribbean contexts, women were key community food providers and agricultural workers, often leading most of the farm labor and land stewardship duties, despite not being able to legally own property and manage farm operations. For example, in the late nineteenth century, Caribbean women's land ownership was based on informal agreements and characterized as unproductive "family land"—leading to women in farming households being redefined as "homemakers," diminishing their roles as "productive" and "gainfully-employed" workers, while individually-owned male land titles and cash crop farming were promoted as legitimate and superior (Green, 2006, p. 17). Relatedly, in African contexts, women farmers played a significant role as the main food providers for their communities, taking on primary tasks of crop production, food processing, and animal husbandry, among others (Ugwu, 2019). Historically, African women were integral to upholding local food systems, making up nearly 50 percent of the agricultural labor in sub-Saharan Africa today; in some contexts, such as Nigeria, they are responsible for up to 80 percent of the farm production labor (Baba et al., 2015).

In the United States, Black women were often the primary food providers for their communities through the early 1900s, leading gardening and farming initiatives for enslaved and sharecropping families.

Later in the twentieth century, Black women served as home demonstration agents as part of the Department of Agriculture's Cooperative Extension service where they led various farming education efforts (Harris, 2009). During the 1960s, Black women were central advocates for food security, agricultural sustainability, and land ownership among collective Black communities, with leaders such as Fannie Lou Hamer emerging as authoritative voices in national conversations on land ownership and community empowerment (McCutcheon, 2019).

Today, ACB women's voice and activism remain on the front lines of emerging mainstream discourse challenging the status quo and transforming the global food landscape toward a just and sustainable future. In the United States, the important public facing work of farmers and grassroots leaders such as Leah Penniman (owner/operator of Soul Fire Farm in Petersburg, New York), Karen Washington (co-owner of Rise and Root Farm in Chester, New York), Gail Taylor (owner of Three-Part Harmony Farm in Washington, D.C.), among other US-based Black women-led food justice groups including National Black Food and Justice Alliance and Patchwork City Farms in Atlanta, Georgia, Feed Our Soul in South Los Angeles, California, and Southeastern African-American Farmers Organic Network (SAAFON) in Decatur, Georgia, have reshaped public discourse around community food security. Black women are also entering into the political arena, with former and current high-ranking officials and Congresswomen, such as Shirley Sherrod, Kim Jackson, Sonya Harper, and Juanita Brent—all agriculturalists in their own right—contributing to conversations recapturing the forgotten legacies of Black women farmers by centering their perspectives in policy discussions on access and sustainability in farming. Similarly, in African and Caribbean contexts, women leaders such as Lilian Nakigozi (founder of Women Smiles in Kampala, Uganda), Wanjiru Kamau-Rutenberg (founder of Akili Dada in Nairobi, Kenya), and Imani Duncan-Price (co-founder of the Caribbean Policy Research Institute in Kingston, Jamaica) have advanced food justice efforts at the policy and community levels. This vast agglomeration of voices has set the foundation for taking ACB women's political voice, lived experience, and cultural knowledge seriously as a catalyst to engender transformative change in agriculture and infuse new directions to the study and practice of food justice and public health.

## [Re]turn to the Community: Foodways, Food Insecurity, and a Critical Reenvisioning of Asset-Based Approaches

Food insecurity is one of the most pressing global health challenges today, impacting 9.9 percent of the world's population, or around 768 million people (FAO, 2022). Defined as a condition where consistent access to adequate food is limited by a lack of money and other resources at times during the year, ACB populations are disproportionately impacted by the condition (Coleman-Jensen et al., 2016). For example, in 2020, over one in five (21.1 percent) US Black households experienced some category of food insecurity—more than three times the rate of their white counterparts (Morales et al., 2020). During the COVID-19 pandemic, Black adults reported the highest rates of food insecurity, with rates 11 percent higher than the national average (Coleman-Jensen et al., 2021). In Caribbean contexts, nearly 40 percent of the population in English-speaking Caribbean countries were food insecure in 2021 (World Bank, 2022). In sub-Saharan African countries, over 66 percent of the population experience moderate-to-severe food insecurity (Wudil et al., 2022). The collective impacts of these inequities have exacerbated global poverty rates, economic instability, social unrest, and migration and displacement, leaving experts in search of ways to stop the proverbial bleeding (Laborde et al., 2020).

Today, prevailing approaches to food insecurity prioritize downstream factors that focus on addressing immediate needs and consumer-level solutions. When food insecurity rates skyrocketed during the COVID-19 pandemic, global health authorities immediately looked to develop and expand on existing food donation and assistance programs. The US government provided $2.76 billion in food assistance to Sub-Saharan Africa in 2022, and $113.68 billion in Supplemental Nutrition Assistance Program emergency allotments to the United States, Guam, and the United States Virgin Islands in 2021 (Congressional Research Service, 2023). Similarly, in 2022, the World Food Programme provided over $3 billion in direct cash assistance to people who are food insecure in seventy-two countries (World Food Programme, 2023). In local and community-based contexts, practitioners often frame food insecurity as an individual-level problem where a lack of education, access, and prohibitive cost are seen as primary contributors, and position behavioral change and food charity models (e.g., food banks, nutrition education programs) as viable solutions (de Souza, 2024; Möller, 2021).

While useful for developing short-term, symptomatic solutions, these approaches do not go far enough in engaging broader structures and root causes, such as prohibitive food and agricultural policies—and, in many ways, reproduce the same inequities they aim to rectify (O'hara & Toussaint, 2021). For example, many charity and food assistance models exist within the private and nonprofit sectors, where they build on market-based logics, such as innovation, efficiency, productivity, and deregulation to address social issues (Broad, 2016; Lohnes & Pine, 2023). Despite their purported benefits, evidence suggests these approaches can create unintended social, cultural, and economic consequences on low-resourced populations deemed "in need" of help (Canfield, 2022). As evidenced, many of these models frame affected communities as passive recipients of proposed interventions by forcing them to rely on the knowledge and resources of outside experts, both in defining problems and articulating relevant solutions (Airhihenbuwa & Dutta, 2012). Moreover, such reliance on market-based mechanisms to develop relevant solutions (e.g., agendas of philanthropically driven campaigns, external grant funders) segments geographic resources and priority funding that silos local and cultural assets, such that transnational cultural meanings around food and land become coopted by development campaigns or erased altogether under the guise of community empowerment and humanitarianism (Dutta, 2020).

Additionally, these models do not document broader cultural, economic, and political contexts, such as how historical trauma and racialized and gendered capitalism inform on-the-ground realities of food insecurity among marginalized communities (Perry & Sealey-Huggins, 2023). Even models that aim to address upstream factors related to food insecurity, such as food production inequities, are often done so under the agreement that local farmers must adopt outside techniques and technologies, in the process erasing localized and context-specific cultural practices, knowledge, and expertise (Adhikari, 2014).

A current snapshot of mainstream public health discourse does not meaningfully address how food insecurity inequities get generated and maintained across higher structural production and distribution processes. More importantly is the missing attention given to unique assets in a community or population, such as *their* capacity to grow and distribute their own food, solve food production disparities, and restore frayed transnational cultural foodways—and the extent to which public health policy can support these efforts. To date, most asset-based models in public health incorporate various "asset mapping" and other participatory approaches to gain a more holistic understanding of community health issues, although the ultimate decision-making power (e.g., program evaluation metrics, allocation of resources, which knowledge "counts") often remains in the hands of the interventionist (Chandanabhumma et al., 2019). More focus is needed on how interventions authentically and equitably identify historical and contemporary cultural and social assets and community connections to food (and land). These omitted perspectives are essential for policymakers and practitioners to develop more just and sustainable food systems that liberate local and global communities, preserve local knowledge and foodways, and meaningfully address multilevel determinants of health among these populations.

Today, a combination of forced displacement, discriminatory policies, and myriad forms of social and economic injustice has largely detached ACB communities from their connection to the land, preventing ACB farmers from meaningfully contributing to the modern agricultural landscape. Nevertheless, there remains a growing number of committed farmers and community advocates to protect ACB cultural farming legacies and collate their shared diasporic knowledge. Extending these perspectives to applied public health contexts, this book introduces NWIAA as a case study to argue that ACB women farmers are vital to suturing fractured ACB foodways and represent new ways to think about emancipatory public policy and health interventions.

## Outline of the Book

*Seeds of Sovereignty* offers an ethnographic investigation into the lived experiences and historical legacies of ACB women farmers, using the community network of NWIAA as a guiding artifact of study. Importantly, the book explores the unique contexts, political strategies, and challenges to mobilizing global ACB women in agriculture and platforming their voices to mainstream audiences. To do so, it draws on the politics of resourcefulness (*POR*; Mackinnon & Derickson, 2013) as a guiding theoretical framework to document the participants' political organizing strategies against the backdrop of intersectional inequity and structural violence. *POR* can be understood as a conceptual praxis "meant to problematize the uneven distribution of material resources and the associated inability of disadvantaged groups and communities to access the levers of social change" (Mackinnon & Derickson, 2013, p. 263). In this way, *POR* "attempts to engage with injustice in terms of both redistribution and recognition toward a vision of resourceful communities, cities and regions" (Mackinnon & Derickson, 2013, p. 263). *POR* offers a theoretical and political critique of how the concept of "resilience" has been applied in social and environmental contexts—suggesting that the term does not critically interrogate existing social relations, is defined by top-down "experts" outside of the targeted communities and is misplaced in terms of spatial scale (e.g., rural, local, regional, global). Rather, *POR* offers "resourcefulness" as a more appropriate concept "to animate politics and activism that seek to transform social relations in more progressive, anti-capitalist and socially just ways" (Mackinnon & Derickson, 2013, p. 255). Opposite of resilience discourses, "resourcefulness as an animating concept specifically seeks to both problematize and redress issues of recognition and redistribution (Fraser, 1996; Young, 1990) and work toward cultivating conditions in which communities can develop alternative visions of social relations" (Mackinnon & Derickson, 2013, p. 255). For interdisciplinary public health practitioners, *POR* is a useful framework for documenting cultural assets and extends a new heuristic for developing upstream community-led and supported intervention models.

Chapter 2 delves more deeply into the book's theoretical underpinnings and relevant scholarly literature, positioning the study within an interdisciplinary axis of Black farming, public health, communication, and social change research. The chapter begins by bringing the reader on a journey to better understand the history of African, Caribbean, and Black (ACB) agricultural inequities in the global food system. Dating back to some of the earliest manifestations, the section threads together diverse scholarship to weave a historical narrative on how these inequities have taken shape over time. Because *Seeds of Sovereignty* takes NWIAA—a US-based organization—as its central case study, the section centers the US food system in this story, providing peripheral context in Africa and the Caribbean along the way. After this landscape is detailed, the second part of the chapter builds on previous scholarship to offer a theoretical and political critique of how "resilience" has been applied in public health interventions and understandings of place and offers *POR* as a more appropriate and just model for public health praxis (Mackinnon & Derickson, 2013). The section begins by establishing "resilience" as the dominant intervention approach to assessing local responses to adverse events, bringing together an interdisciplinary discussion around the concept. Next, the section interrogates assumptive logics that undergird these models by foregrounding scholarly criticisms that highlight the shortcomings of such approaches. Finally, the section introduces *POR* as the book's guiding theoretical framework.

Chapters 3 to 5 comprise the book's research findings. The third chapter situates the specific study context and establishes the current social and political conditions for ACB women farmers. The chapter opens with an oral history of NWIAA's executive director and founder, Tammy Gray-Steele, and her family's unique entry point into agriculture. The narrative underscores some of the current challenges ACB farmers face and brings attention to Black futurist imaginings of land ownership and community sovereignty given different social and political circumstances. Building on this story, the chapter moves to the present to explore how the featured women of NWIAA describe the diverse relational barriers they experienced when navigating dominant agricultural spaces. This context is important for documenting the cumulative impact of on-the-ground, micro-forms of inequity that ACB women endure and complicating dominant narratives that frame access as the primary determinant to fostering equity.

Chapter 4 documents how the women navigated structural inequities while protecting and advancing their cultural legacies and shared deep-rooted agricultural knowledge by applying two axioms of *POR*, *resources* and *recognition*, to the corpus of ethnographic data. The first part of the chapter explores how participants discussed *resources* as a *POR* strategy, drawing specific attention to how they created material and discursive conditions to come together, "take up" physical and intellectual space, cultivate alternative communication infrastructures, and forge weak-tie partnerships within systems of oppression that were set up to disenfranchise them. The second part documents the resourcefulness strategies participants used to engender external and internal *recognition* from both top-down power brokers and in-group community stakeholders, and how these actions were constrained by the complex sociopolitical conditions that undergirded them.

Chapter 5 spans beyond participants' microlevel realities and observations to document how they discussed alternative ways of knowing and practices around land, food, and agriculture and transformative visions for food system and public health change by applying a third POR axiom, *indigenous and folk knowledge*, to the corpus of data. The chapter highlights the participants' reflections as they aligned across the primary themes of people-place connections, cultural heritage, and futurist imaginings.

Chapter 6 concludes the book, summarizing the key theoretical, empirical, and methodological contributions. The featured case study highlights how NWIAA employed resourcefulness strategies in their efforts to protect ACB food and farming legacies and promote community food security. Nonetheless, it documents how the organization's mobilizing strategies were limited by broader political barriers, interorganizational ambivalence, and underlying race, gender, and class tensions, complicating the possibilities of multi-sector organizing to support ACB community sovereignty. The chapter discusses the implications of the book's findings for interdisciplinary health, agriculture, and social justice research; it also ponders the future possibilities of ACB farming and public health interventions against the backdrop of the current social and political climate.

## A Note on Methods and Positionality

Before bringing this introduction to a close, it is important to detail the methodological approach that guided this study, including my individual standpoint and positionality as a researcher. The study design builds on principles of critical ethnography (Madison, 2011). This framework is a participatory approach to research that explicitly sets out to critique hegemony, oppression, and asymmetrical power relations to promote social change (Palmer & Caldas, 2015). Given the study's focus on centering ACB women farmers' voices and how they describe power inequities and structural violence in agriculture and public health, the guiding tenets of critical ethnography are particularly well-suited to interrogate these concepts deeply. I used four primary data collection methods throughout the study: semi-structured interviews, observations, surveys, and participatory action research activities.

Participants engaged in two separate interviews. During the first interview, participants were asked questions about their farming background and personal identity, their lived experiences as an ACB woman farmer, and their involvement with NWIAA. The second interview comprised questions that were drawn from tenets of *POR*; interview guide themes included questions about cultural heritage, resources (e.g., community networks and infrastructure), people-place connections, recognition, and alternative knowledge. All interviews took place via Zoom video conferencing software; this medium was strategically selected to ensure the best sound quality for audio recording and transcription and minimize extraneous noise common in natural research settings. A total of twenty-nine people (twenty-seven women, two men) participated in the study.

I engaged in formal and informal observations throughout the duration of the ethnographic project. Observations took place across a wide range of settings and contexts, including in-person at NWIAA's Veterans Women in Agriculture Conference, fifteenth Year Anniversary Celebration (both held in Oklahoma City, Oklahoma), National Women in Agriculture Conference (held in Compton, California), Equity and Inclusion March and invited White House meeting (both held in Washington, D.C.), USVI field site visit (held in St. Croix, USVI), and virtually at NWIAA's annual training workshops, meeting with former United States Deputy Secretary of Agriculture Jewel Bronaugh, and NWIAA Africa monthly chapter leader meetings. Some of my primary observation activities included: individual hand-written and digital field notes, audio-recorded voice memos, taking photographs and videos. I used discernible caution when engaging in observations, making sure to do so only when it was deemed appropriate and did not interrupt the natural research setting.

The third form of data collection was descriptive surveys. Before participating in the semi-structured interview, participants were asked to fill out a short sociodemographic survey via Qualtrics experience management software. The survey included questions about the participants' gender, race/ethnicity, education level, employment status, country of origin, farm size, and types of crop(s) grown. The goal of the survey was to triangulate the robust qualitative findings and offer descriptive data to support the lived realities and challenges participants experienced. For instance, one insightful finding of the survey was that 45 percent of respondents' farm size was less than five acres, drawing attention to both the impressive determination and community organizing capacity the women were able to generate, given their dearth of resources and their perceived limited political power as small-scale farmers.

I also engaged in several participatory action research activities throughout the project. This data collection method is different than observations in that it involves collaborative engagement and activism between researcher and participants to identify a problem, develop solutions, and implement actions. During the project, I actively participated in a diversity of activities and served different roles with the organization, including political ally, advisor, and community partner. For example, during the Equity and Inclusion protest in Washington DC, I marched in solidarity with the participants via police escort from the US Capitol building to the White House and offered a testimonial on behalf of the organization on the White House lawn. During NWIAA's invited White House visit to meet with administration staffers to discuss their proposal to become a congressionally chartered organization and serve as a pilot program of 4-H (a US-based network of organizations that develop citizenship, leadership, responsibility, and life skills of youth through experiential learning and a positive youth development approach) for Black youth in agriculture, NWIAA leadership asked me to provide testimony on their behalf, where I used my published academic research to demonstrate the organization's effectiveness in addressing community food security, mobilizing Black women farmers, and engaging Black youth in agriculture. In addition, I contributed expertise as an advisor by drawing on my journalism training to draft/edit press releases, speech transcripts, correspondence emails, grant proposals, in addition to "power-sharing" by bringing their stories to dominant communication platforms (e.g., research journals, academic conferences, national op-eds) and helping craft rhetorically persuasive messages to external stakeholders.

Lastly, reflecting on my research positionality and standpoint is important given the critically oriented nature of this study. The term positionality refers to both a researcher's worldview and the stance they adopt in relation to their scholarly investigations and relevant social and political context (Holmes, 2020). In recent years, calls for researchers to document their positionality and its role in influencing the process and outcomes of research have become more frequent, particularly in the social science and humanistic fields that account for the subjective nature of research. For critical scholars, documenting positionality is also important for illuminating power differentials and privilege and marginalization spaces as they exist between researcher and community.

I do not write *Seeds of Sovereignty* from a socially or politically neutral position and have arrived at this research on account of several deep personal and academic experiences. My passion and interest in food and health justice was first ignited after witnessing firsthand my mother's lifelong struggle with diabetes and associated challenges navigating a cumbersome and confusing health care system that largely exacerbated her condition. When she ultimately passed away from the condition after years of what I would characterize as health communication discordances at best—a form of neglect and potential malpractice at worst—I became motivated to explore how the structural barriers rife in our health care system impact individual quality-of-care and health outcomes. These experiences ultimately led me to pursue a doctoral degree in critical health communication, a field that interrogates how things like power dynamics, cultural contexts, social inequities, and structural factors shape health-related communication processes and outcomes. My combined scholarly training and applied background in public health provided the intellectual foundation for this project.

My entry point to this research is also informed by my multiple social identities, which granted me emic (or insider) perspectives to the research context in some situations, and etic (or outsider) perspectives in others (Creswell, 1998). I grew up in a two-parent, multiracial household with a Black father and white mother in Southern California, where deep engagements on topics such as race and racism were common. My father's side of the family has roots in the US South, specifically Alabama, where we have direct linkages to the same racialized histories of labor and Black southern foodways documented in this book. I also come from a lineage of strong and pioneering Black women who have profoundly shaped my worldview on race and gender and instilled in me a deep sense of humility when engaging with my research participants.

My middle-class upbringing has afforded me certain privileges that influenced how I approached the research for this book. For example, I have never experienced food insecurity or fear of going hungry. This social location positioned me as an outsider in relation to understanding how individuals who are food insecure experience food system inequities and ecological challenges. My positionality as an academic and college professor gave me access to important social resources and the analytical tools, expertise, and credibility to serve as a political ally; however, my doctoral training gave me etic perspectives in relation to the specific study context.

By reflexively interrogating my positionality, my goal is to be transparent about how my background, identity, and lived experiences intersect with the study. This practice, I hope, will foster accountability and enhance the rigor and overall validity of this research.

# 2

## How Did We Get Here?

### Situating Agricultural Inequities in the Food System and Interrogating Resilience

IN *SEEDS OF SOVEREIGNTY*, I highlight African, Caribbean, and Black women farmers' historical lived experiences, political voices, and deep-rooted agricultural expertise to motivate readers to radically re-envision how we collectively organize our public health and food systems. Importantly, I levy a range of critiques against dominant approaches to "doing" food security interventions, suggesting that an overreliance on downstream and individual-level solutions (e.g., education and awareness campaigns, survey self-reporting methodologies) and working within existing status quo structural configurations (e.g., farm subsidy and geographic zoning policies) clouds practitioners vision from thinking holistically about ways to address root causes—which are often artificially created and upheld by broader inequities in the food system. These injustices, further reinforced by structures of capitalism and government deregulation, segment resources and promote an uneven funding landscape that support certain cause—effect rationales while simultaneously siloing expertise in how problems are defined and solutions generated (for example, defining food insecurity as solely within

*Seeds of Sovereignty*. Andrew L. Carter, Oxford University Press. © Oxford University Press (2026).
DOI: 10.1093/9780197789391.003.0002

the parameters of "public health" with limited cross-pollinated contributions from sectors such as agriculture, public policy, and urban/rural planning). To paint a more accurate picture of how ACB food inequities have come to be today requires a synergistic approach that accounts for the combined insults across public health, to include agricultural history as a way to identify structural root causes and document overlooked cultural and social assets. This chapter brings together some of this necessary context.

The chapter unfolds across two primary sections. The first part brings the reader on a journey to better understand the history of ACB agricultural inequities in the global food system. Dating back to some of the earliest manifestations, the section threads together interdisciplinary scholarship to weave a historical narrative on how these inequities have taken shape over time. Given the US-centricity of National Women in Agriculture Association (NWIAA) and the study context, the section centers the US food system in this story, providing supporting context in Africa and the Caribbean along the way. After this context is detailed, the second part of the chapter builds on previous scholarship to offer a theoretical and political critique of how "resilience" has been applied in public health interventions and understandings of place and offers politics of resourcefulness (*POR*) as a more appropriate and just model for public health praxis (Mackinnon & Derickson, 2013). The section begins by establishing "resilience" as the dominant intervention approach to assessing local responses to adverse events, bringing together an interdisciplinary discussion around the concept. Next, the section interrogates assumptive logics that undergird these models by collating several scholarly criticisms that highlight the shortcomings of such approaches. Finally, the section introduces *POR* as the book's guiding theoretical framework.

## African, Caribbean, and Black Agricultural Inequities in the Global Food System

Today's global food landscape reflects a stark binary between those who have access to high-quality, culturally appropriate, nutritious food and those who do not; though this current snapshot does not exist without context, and situates within intersecting social, historical, political, economic, and cultural dimensions. Centuries of discriminatory policies, land and knowledge theft, cultural erasure, and overt violence have shaped current on-the-ground contexts that unduly impact transnational ACB communities across all levels of the food system. Drawing on the understanding that addressing broader historical inequities in the food system would drastically improve diasporic ACB food security and health outcomes, it is essential to pinpoint the genesis of these inequities and how they have transformed over time.

## Tracing the Origins: From Colonialism to Slavery and Reconstruction (Early 1500s–1870)

The initial catalyst responsible for disassembling African foodways and farming techniques and spearheading many of today's global food and health inequities began during the early 1500s, when European colonizers invaded Africa to dramatically upend all aspects of collective African societies, including how they organized their food systems (De Zwart & Van Zanden, 2018; Parker & Rathbone, 2007; Widgren, 2017). For African agrarian communities, this shift had widespread consequences that disrupted their traditional farming practices and altered land ownership structures and local economies (Raschke & Cheema, 2008; Waites, 2005). Prior to colonization, these communities cultivated a wide range of indigenous crops suited to their regional climates, soils, and ecosystems, and supported local trade economies and agricultural practices (Beinart, 2000). Drawing on centuries of local knowledge and cultural context, the farmers were responsible for pioneering a range of innovative sustainable agricultural practices. For example, many modern forms of polyculture, intercropping, and agroforestry have foundational roots in West African farming traditions[1] (Mapara, 2009). However, European colonization displaced many of

[1] Many of these traditional African practices are still widely used today and recognized by leaders in environmental sustainability and alternative food arenas as effective solutions to address climate change, mitigate food insecurity, and create more resilient food systems; though many African nations are not properly recognized for their contribution in creating these techniques and upholding this legacy (Penniman, 2018; 2022).

these innovations by introducing cash-crop economies to the region, which prioritized growing commodity crops such as sugar, cotton, and tobacco that could maximize profits on the global market and were positioned as superior to "primitive" and inefficient African food systems (Parker & Rathbone, 2007). In places like Nigeria and Ghana, these once agrarian-based economies would become catalysts for a growing global cocoa and palm oil industry (Austin, 2009).

This hegemonic shift would slowly begin to erase Indigenous African cultural connections to land and traditional foodways (Roessler et al., 2020; 2022). Processes of colonization also introduced Western farming techniques to the African region, which, despite their capacity to maximize yields, were largely incompatible with local environments and growing conditions (Beinart & Hughes, 2007). For instance, early practices of monocropping (a farming method where a single crop is grown on the same land without rotating other crops) were implemented to support the level of large-scale farming required to meet cash-crop demands, yet they were responsible for a host of negative environmental impacts, such as soil depletion, increased pest and disease vulnerability, loss of biodiversity, and reduced crop resilience (Sousa & Raizada, 2020). Of course, these transgressions emerged alongside more insidious and overt forms of violence, such as stealing vast areas of fertile African land to establish farm plantations, displacing Indigenous communities from their ancestral lands, and the imposition of new tax systems meant to socially marginalize and politically disenfranchise local African communities (Jalata, 2013).

As cash-crop economies grew into the late 1500s, the availability of cheap and accessible labor became paramount for European colonial powers to maintain and expand large-scale production into new markets. In response, European colonizers initiated the transatlantic slave trade to meet this rising demand, which had particularly devastating impacts for both Indigenous and diasporic African farming populations. As millions of farmers were forcibly removed to supply the Western labor demand, exiting with them were their unique agricultural skillsets, traditional farming practices, and contributions to their local economies (Fields-Black, 2008; Littlefield, 1991). This involuntary brain drain left many African regions vulnerable to famine, economic decline, and ruptured food systems that reproduced widespread social inequity.

Meanwhile, on the receiving end of this labor, plantation owners in places like the United States and the Caribbean benefited extensively from Africans' extensive agricultural expertise and farming knowledge, which they harnessed to improve the productivity of cash crops. For example, in the US South in places like South Carolina and Georgia, large-scale rice and cotton cultivation relied heavily on knowledge practices of slaves from Senegal and Cameroon relating to irrigation, seed selection, soil management techniques, pest control, and plant breeding (Carney, 2001; Jordan, 2013; Robins, 2016). In the Caribbean, particularly in places like St. Croix and the West Indies, plantation owners drew extensively from the agricultural expertise of enslaved Angola, Nigeria, and Ghana to grow and process sugarcane—a cornerstone of the region's economy (Halcrow, 1982; Thurland, 2014). Over the course of the next few hundred years, ACB farmers were systematically co-opted for their unique and innovative agricultural skillsets while simultaneously being further distanced from their cultural connection to indigenous lands, which created a legacy of exploitation and environmental and public health degradation that persisted long after the subsequent abolition of slavery.

In the US, the official abolishment of chattel slavery ended with the Emancipation Proclamation towards the end of the Civil War in 1863. Though for Black American farmers, the Reconstruction period that followed birthed a new set of inequities that reverberated transnationally to impact diasporic communities. As the US grappled with the question of how to integrate millions of newly freed Black Americans into existing social, political, and labor systems, several constitutional amendments and Reconstruction Acts were developed by Union lawmakers in response to facilitate this transition (Foner, 1988). Among these efforts, one proposed solution—the "40 acres and a mule" mandate—had the potential to meaningfully address centuries of endured slave labor, structural violence, agricultural knowledge and culture co-optation (Reid & Bennett, 2012). Initially promised to Black freedmen on January 16, 1865, as a part of Special Field Orders #15, the legislative order, spearheaded by former Union General William T. Sherman in consultation with a select group of Black ministers, divided 40,000 acres of former slave plantations into small farm plots as a reparative action to foster Black economic freedom and self-sufficiency (Darity Jr., 2008).

Despite the mandate's transformative potential, its short-lived promise was over before it began. Following the assassination of Abraham Lincoln, a few months later on April 15, 1865, Andrew Johnson succeeded to the presidency and immediately reversed Sherman's Field Orders #15—returning much of the 400,000 re-allocated acres back to Southern landowners. Few Black families were able to take advantage of the mandate, and the landmark decision to redact the order represented one of the last opportunities for large-scale land reform to take place in the US. Johnson's legacy of racist governance would continue in subsequent years when he enacted the Black Codes, a series of laws designed to limit the economic, social, and political freedom of newly freed Black Americans and ensure the maintenance of a plantation economy for decades to come in the antebellum South. The Black Codes were responsible for limiting Black voting and legal rights, job opportunities, property ownership, and instituting vagrancy laws.

For Black farmers specifically, the combined redaction of the "40 acres" mandate and legalized Black Codes had a devastating and enduring impact on their agricultural legacy. For example, without land of their own to farm, many freedmen were left with no choice but to work as sharecroppers and tenant farmers on the very land promised to them months prior, setting up generational legacies of trauma, poverty, and financial debt. These challenges were made worse by documents of direct violence and intimidation from hate groups such as the Ku Klux Klan, restricted access to educational opportunities and training resources due to discriminatory policies and the gross underfunding of many 1890 Black land grant universities, and racist lending practices that made acquiring additional land and becoming competitive in the agriculture landscape nearly impossible (Olsen, 1962).

Mirroring trends on the US mainland, similar trajectories were happening in parts of the Caribbean that saw newly freed Black Caribbeans experience temporary emancipation, only to be followed by new forms of legislation that relegated them back to servitude. For example, slavery in the Danish West Indies (which would become the US Virgin Islands after the US purchased the territory from Denmark in 1917) was provisionally abolished in 1848 after a combination of British and French abolitionist movements, the declining profitability of plantation economies, and various resistance movements and revolts spearheaded it's cessation (Tomich, 2016). However, similar to

President Johnson's response in the US, this newfound freedom was fleeting. In the time immediately following emancipation, many freed Black Caribbeans "basked in long-desired idleness and flatly refused to work," which set off a growing chorus of plantation owner gripes about challenges towards re-establishing a reliable labor force with enslaved workers (Harrigan & Varlack, 1977, p. 392). Within months of emancipation, strict legislation was passed to mitigate the immediate and large-scale labor loss. Known as the Labor Act of 1849,[2] the legislation was similar to the "vagrancy laws" associated with Johnson's Black Codes in the US and would once again uphold the plantation economy for subsequent years in the region (Marsh, 1981).

This institutional labor setting would engender a range of deleterious consequences for Black Caribbean farmers. For example, the Labor Act grossly favored the interests of the plantation elite, which gave them ultimate negotiating power over labor contracts (Theodoridis et al., 2024). As freedmen were required by law to enter into contracts with plantation owners, they were forced to accept unfairly low wages that preserved class inequities and limited their capacity to accumulate land and wealth (Galli et al., 2024). The Act also placed constraints on freedmen's ability to grow their own "subsistence plots"[3] and maintain their cultural foodways.

## Sowing New Injustice: Jim Crow, The Great Depression, and The Promise of a Black Farming Renaissance (Late 1870s–1960s)

The decades following Reconstruction brought forth a host of new challenges for ACB farmers that set off a cascade of separate but interrelated transgressional events negatively impacting global diasporic

[2] The Labor Act of 1849 required freedmen in the USVI to remain working on the same plantations under strict labor contracts, limiting their ability to seek other employment. The Act relegated former slaves to indentured servitude with low wages and harsh working conditions. The legislation provided the planter elite with access to a cheap and reliable labor force.

[3] A common practice among plantation owners in the Caribbean was to provide slaves with their own micro-plots of land, commonly referred to as "subsistence plots" as a means for them to grow food to feed themselves and maximize profits. These micro-plots also provided slave communities with a sense of independence and allowed them to preserve some of their farming techniques and cultural foodways (Edmonstone, 2024). However, most of these informal land agreements were prohibited after the Labor Act (McKittrick, 2013).

communities. As systems of sharecropping became entrenched in the US South as the "predominant capital-labor arrangement" between vulnerable and impoverished freedmen and exploitative white elite landowners, Black farmers would enter a new era of racial repression that relegated them to indentured servitude (Riddle, 1995, p. 53). Though technically free to move about at their own will as newly legal citizens, the iniquitous systems of sharecropping kept many Black farmers bound to peonage agreements and forced labor in many of the same ways that slavery did (Hinson & Robinson, 2008). More importantly, the agreements were responsible for burdening Black farmers with perpetually increasing debts and limited access to legal support, which ensured they had no ownership of the land or what it produced (Hinson & Robinson, 2008). These challenges emerged against the backdrop of a bevy of other discriminatory legislative actions, including the Civil Rights Act of 1883 (which effectively struck down the Civil Rights Act of 1875) and subsequent Jim Crow laws, which ushered in a "separate-but-equal" mandate that would take hold until the mid-twentieth century.

In the wake of these multitudinous challenges, Black farmers determinably developed an array of innovative strategies to share resources and build out their capacities to farm independently—some of which included leveraging and preserving the limited resources provided to them by the Freedman's Bureau directly following the Civil War,[4] saving money through sharecropping to eventually buy small plots of land, and relying on limited access to credit from Black-owned institutions and the increasing willingness of some white landowners to sell directly to Black farmers (Copeland, 1984). Notably, during this time, many Black farmers banded together to form cooperatives, which allowed them to purchase seeds and supplies without relying on predatory lenders and pool their shared knowledge, best practices, and economic resources (Reynolds, 2002). These combined efforts cultivated a Black farming renaissance in the US; in 1920, Black farmers owned between

[4] The Freedman's Bureau was a US government agency that provided newly freed slaves access to education, legal assistance, and labor contracts, food, shelter, and, in some cases, land. The services helped freedmen transition to freedom and gain economic independence.

16 and 19 million acres of farmland and represented 14 percent of the national farming population (Gilbert et al., 2002).

Unfortunately, this short-lived moment of Black agricultural prosperity did not last long, as the end of the decade was bookended by the worst economic downturn in the history of the industrialized world: The Great Depression. While the financial crisis impacted all aspects of global society, it was particularly devastating for the US farming population. A combination of falling farm product prices, crop surpluses, a crumbling national banking system, and decreased overall spending saw around 45 percent of farms face foreclosure by 1933 (Hausman et al., 2021). To mitigate these encompassing crises, President Franklin Delano Roosevelt passed the Agricultural Adjustment Act (AAA) in 1933 as a part of his New Deal legislative efforts as a bailout action to support the country's struggling farmers. The key goal of the AAA was to increase crop prices by reducing surpluses and limiting production. As part of the Act, the government offered subsidies to farmers in exchange for not planting certain crops and purchased livestock for slaughter to address oversupply concerns.

Indeed, the AAA was moderately successful in rescuing the American agriculture industry from immediate collapse and providing significant relief to many farmers; however, the legislation had devastating consequences for the country's Black farming population. To begin, many of Roosevelt's New Deal policies were implemented in ways that favored landowners (which were almost exclusively white), leaving Black farmers with little control over agricultural policy decisions and limited direct access to financial assistance. Even when the USDA tried to implement farm loan programs to help farm tenants, laborers, and sharecroppers purchase land and other necessary farming resources through the Bankhead-Jones Farm Tenant Act in 1937, they were largely decentralized and left ultimate decision-making power for determining farm loan lending decisions to designated local county committees—who were mostly affluent white landowners with incentives to maintain the status quo (Reid, 2007; Tyler & Moore, 2013). Additionally, AAA's focus on limiting overall crop production incentivized many landowners to take their land out of production to reduce surpluses and become eligible for government subsidy payments. As a part of this strategy, the landowners often eliminated sharecropping and tenant farming arrangements altogether, which saw many Black farmers get evicted from their homes and deemed ineligible to receive social benefits and their own subsidies (Depew et al., 2013). These collective obstacles, which included other systemic inequities like the rife discrimination embedded in New Deal—era public works programs such as the Resettlement Administration, were responsible for setting up an entrenched racial order in agriculture that remained obstinate to change for years to come (Carroll, 2014; Folsom Jr., 2009). More impactfully, FDR's farm subsidy programs laid the seeds for the large-scale, multinational, corporatized global food system of today.

Though not directly impacted by the systemic inequities brought forth by the US post-Reconstruction sharecropping agreements or the exclusionary policies embedded in the AAA, global ACB farming communities experienced parallel instantiations of oppression and violence. For example, in Kenya, the British were responsible for displacing indigenous farming communities as part of their White Highlands land theft in the early twentieth century. The region, located in Central Kenya, was known historically for its ideal farming conditions, fertile volcanic soil, and a foundational hub for Kenyan communities to preserve their traditional foodways and local food systems. However, under British colonial rule, much of the region's roughly seven million acres of highly fertile land was directly stolen from Indigenous Kenyans as part of the Crown Lands Ordinances of 1902 and 1915. The policies declared that all land in Kenya, except for that which was already privately owned, was considered "Crown Land" and under control of the British government, and was used to ensure the region was reserved exclusively for European settlers (Morgan, 1963). Local Kenyans, meanwhile, were forcibly removed from their ancestral lands and mandated to live on smaller, overcrowded reserves with less arable land plots. The Crown Lands Ordinances represented another node in a complex, interconnected history of ACB farming communities' forced removal from land and destruction of transnational foodways. Far from an isolated example, other African farming communities across the continent experienced similar forms of land theft and cultural violence during the early to mid-1900s.[5]

Black Caribbean farmers faced their own set of unique challenges during the time that birthed similar, albeit less direct, forms of displacement and cultural erasure. In the USVI, the bourgeoning sugarcane economy—which represented a central junction in the triangular molasses trade—began to falter in the mid-twentieth century due to overall declines in sugar prices, labor shortages, and increased productivity due to mechanization. After the region's last sugar mill, the Estate Diamond Mill, officially closed its doors in 1966, it marked the end of its global influence in agriculture, to which political leadership began to shift its focus to tourism (Gruver et al., 2024). In many ways, this economic transition signaled the end of Black Caribbean farmers' regional legacy in agriculture and the food system dating back to slavery. As the sugar industry failed, many farmers did not know how to transition to growing other crops, and development projects overtook the land that previous generations had used for farming, rather than safeguarding it for agricultural use (Blaut et al., 1965). Simultaneously, the tourism industry afforded opportunities for seasonally employed workers and was seen as more lucrative than working in agriculture for many Black Caribbean farmers. However, this shift in the economy did not come without consequence. For example, between 1790 and 1960, the USVI produced most of the food it consumed (Crossman et al., 2010). However, a combination of the waning agriculture industry and proximity of the region to other island nations and the US provided easy access to cheap, readily available foods; by the 1980s, the USVI was importing 99 percent of the food its populous consumed—a statistic that is still true today (Gruver et al., 2024). This combined shift contributed to the continued erasure of ACB foodways in the region and fostered a forced reliance on the dominant food system.

[5] Other related examples of African farmers' erasure and land theft include the Land Apportionment Act of 1930 in Zimbabwe, the Natives' Land Act of 1913 and Native Trust and Land Act of 1936 in South Africa, and the *Chibalo* system of debt bondage and forced labor in Portuguese Angola and Mozambique through the mid-1900s.

## [Un]just Fields and "Broken Promises": ACB Agricultural Inequities in the Modern Era (1980s–Today)

In recent decades, ACB agriculture inequities have been upheld and made worse by existing policies and strategic political decisions designed to ensure status quo relationships and dominance hierarchies in the food system. As the initial insults of European colonization and subsequent centuries of direct violence and subjugation created the landscape for vast injustice, the careful construction of the modern food system has worked to cement these social conditions into reality. This manifestation has taken shape in different forms and contexts for ACB diasporic farmers.

In the US, several factors have led to this current reality, including the mechanization of agriculture and increases in technology (that outpriced many Black farmers from participating in the field), the erasure of ACB farming traditions, cultural shifts away from farming into other professions, among others (Carter & Alexander, 2020; Reynolds, 2002; Wood & Ragar, 2012). However, arguably the biggest catalyst behind today's inequitable landscape for Black farmers is the endless array of transgressions on the part of the US Department of Agriculture. While initial grievances of Black farmer discrimination were first documented dating back to the 1960s, the 1980s and 90s were particularly rampant with rife injustice across ecological contexts (Hayes, 2021). For example, in 1982, a report from the US Commission of Civil Rights titled "The Decline of Black Farming in America" was one of the first comprehensive government documents that directly identified racial discrimination as a key factor in the decline of Black farmers (which fell to 2% earlier that year). The following year, in 1983, citing budget cuts, President Ronald Reagan disbanded the USDA Office of Civil Rights and stopped responding to claims of discrimination—which was reflective of the level of disregard the government had for meaningfully addressing Black farmer injustices (US Government Accountability Office, 2008). Prior to its removal, the Office played a key role in enforcing civil rights laws, ensuring nondiscrimination in programs administered by the USDA, and addressing complaints and instances of discrimination faced by Black farmers, particularly regarding access to credit and assistance necessary for sustaining and expanding their agricultural operations (Sinclair, 1984).

During the 1990s, a series of public and private reports from key interest groups and political leaders detailed wide-ranging discrimination around the unequal access to programs (e.g., farm subsidy payments, disaster relief, technical assistance), denial of farm loans, local forms of collusion and bias (e.g., USDA county committee system), and direct forms of retaliation and intimidation against Black farmers. Ultimately, this led to the USDA participating in one of the largest civil rights settlements in US history: the 1999 Pigford v. Glickman class action lawsuit. The $1.03 billion settlement[6] was a direct admission of guilt in acknowledging the government's failure to treat Black farmers equitably in administering farm loans, grants, and assistance programs. Though a promising first step, significant flaws in implementation marked by red tape barriers saw many eligible farmers not receive payments (only 15,645 out of 22,000 farmers received modest payments, and only 2,585 of over 61,000 late claims were accepted).[7]

Much of the twenty-first century has been marked by worsening disparities between Black and white farmers and increased forms of direct and indirect discrimination. In addition to the vast decline in the Black farming population overall (in 2002, the Black farmer rate fell to 1.3 percent, where it has relatively remained over the past two decades), exacerbating disparities in farm subsidy allocations persist. For instance, in 2002, Black farmers received $21.2 million in farm subsidies, while white farmers received $8.9 billion; in 2007, these disparities expanded to $38 million and $10.6 billion, respectively, drawing attention to deep-seated inequities in inherited wealth and credit to purchase land. The past decade has brought about various efforts and legislative actions

---

[6] Eligible farmers in the original Pigford lawsuit were awarded $50,000 each along with debt relief and tax offsets.

[7] In 2008, a second lawsuit (the "Pigford II" case) was initiated, which was an extension of the original Pigford v. Glickman settlement. The case addressed further claims of racial discrimination by Black farmers who were excluded from the initial settlement, providing them new opportunities to seek compensation if they could prove they were unfairly denied loans or assistance based on their race between 1981 and 1996.

to address these inequities, though they have not led to any meaningful policy legislation. For example, the Justice for Black Farmers Act (JBFA)[8] was a legislative proposal introduced in the US Senate in 2021 by Senators Cory Booker, Elizabeth Warren, and Kirsten Gillibrand that aimed to address head-on the historical and systemic discrimination of the USDA and support the revitalization of Black-owned farms and land ownership. Despite its transformative potential, the bill was never passed into law and currently sits idly in a nebulous state.

Other, more ambitious efforts to address Black farmer inequities were strongly opposed and fervently struck down by the government and general public alike. For example, President Biden's Emergency Relief for Farmers of Color Act (ERFCA) was signed into law on August 16, 2021, but was repealed after several white farmers filed lawsuits to block it, arguing that the federal government was engaging in reverse discrimination by awarding money based on race (Levenson, 2021). The lawsuits were spearheaded by America Legal First, a conservative public interest organization with direct ties to the President Trump administration. The ERFCA would have been one of the largest pieces of legislation for Black farmers to date (Reiley, 2021). To mitigate the public backlash, the federal government created two additional funding streams to help farmers as part of the revised Inflation Reduction Act (a $2.2 billion program for farmers who faced discrimination prior to 2021, and a separate $3.1 billion program to cover loans for farmers facing financial distress, particularly against the social circumstances of COVID-19). While the latter program has paid $2.2 billion to more than 40,000 people, the former has not yet initiated any payments; further, it took focus off Black farmers exclusively to include farmers from all ethnic groups. Many Black farmer leaders deemed this a "broken promise" reflective of a larger history of government betrayal, leading

[8] The Justice for Black Farmers Act (JBFA) was a marker bill included in the 2023 US Farm Bill. Key goals of the JBFA included ending discrimination in the USDA by creating an independent civil rights oversight board and equity commission, protecting Black farmer land loss and restoring their land base, providing resources to land grant HBCUs, and assisting socially disadvantaged farmers and ranchers (Congress.gov, 2023).

a group of them to file a class-action countersuit against the federal government (McFetridge, 2022).

More recently, in 2022, the USDA invested $3.1 billion in 141 selected projects under the Partnerships for Climate-Smart Commodities program, an initiative aimed to expand markets for climate-smart commodities and "provide direct, meaningful benefits to production agriculture, including for small and underserved producers." The initiative was meant to support "a diverse range of farmers, ranchers, and private forest landowners," though the leading partners from projects with the largest funding ceilings (i.e., $70M–$95M; $50M–$65M) were predominately white and from large-scale corporations, such as PepsiCo, Coca Cola, Cargill, Microsoft, Hershey, Keurig-Dr. Pepper, and John Deere. Funded projects that *did* incorporate representation from Black farmer-led organizations and other marginalized communities were from the smallest funding ceilings (i.e., $25000–under $5M; $5M–$20M) and often engaged such groups in a participatory capacity (a model often employed by top-down power brokers to leverage the trust and rooted authenticity of such groups to garner community buy-in and gain a more holistic understanding of on-the-ground issues and contexts, although they ultimate control decision-making power, including program evaluation metrics, allocation of resources, and which data "count" as relevant and impactful). These collective impacts have worked to uphold the glaringly inequitable landscape for Black farmers in the US.

In African contexts, the modern era of agriculture has shuttled in new forms of inequity that have exacerbated the cascading erasure of ACB foodways and farming practices globally. Notably, the central vehicle for much of these transgressions has come in the form of "problematizing" African farming economies as primitive and in need of external intervention, creating pathways for an increased reliance on West-centric agricultural innovation efforts (that mirrored some of the same cultural logics and subversive tactics as their colonial past). This strategy was largely carried out in the form of privatizing seed and agricultural input markets. For example, following a number of global economic shocks in the 1970s that catalyzed a rapid decline in commodity prices and worsening trade conditions for Sub-Saharan African (SSA) countries, the region became a focal point for the implementation of Structural Adjustment Programs[9] introduced by the International Monetary Fund and the World Bank.[10] The programs were positioned as a way to provide financial assistance and debt relief to fragile African economies and promote development; they were instituted in over forty SSA countries throughout the 1980s and 90s (Heidhues & Obare, 2011). While the programs were marginally effective in providing short-term economic relief for some SSA countries, they had broader social and political consequences that negatively impacted global ACB foodways and farming communities (Abah & Naankiel, 2016; Crisp & Kelly, 1999). As these models were built upon principles of austerity and economic efficiency, they were carried out by incorporating neoliberal practices such as privatizing state-controlled industries (e.g., seed companies and agricultural input suppliers), reducing state support (e.g., subsidies for agriculture, extension services, and rural development), and promoting trade liberalization and agricultural exports (e.g., cash-crop production). This created an environment rife for multinational corporations to overtake control of global markets via patented seed and other agricultural innovations, while concurrently diminishing local biodiversity and ACB knowledge systems.

African farmers' forced reliance on external agricultural innovation was intensified in the following decades when the international non-profit Alliance for a Green Revolution (AGRA; a partnership between the Bill and Melinda Gates Foundation and the Rockefeller

---

[9] Structural Adjustment Programs are economic reform policies imposed on developing countries, requiring austerity measures, market liberalization, and privatization in exchange for loans or debt restructuring.

[10] The world economic turmoil in the 1970s was largely a result of a breakdown in the Bretton Woods system of fixed exchange rates and gold convertibility of the United States dollar, two oil price shocks, and stagflation (e.g., a rare economic condition characterized by the simultaneous occurrence of high inflation, stagnant economic growth, and elevated unemployment) that weakened the economies of many developed countries. This caused a decline in commodity prices and a deterioration of trade for many developing countries whose main exports were commodities. Ironically, the dominance of commodity markets in most SSA countries first came about when they were forced to be adopted during European colonization in the 1500s. This economic "problematization" was an example of West-centric power brokers constructing a problem so that they can create a market to "fix" it.

Foundation) invested roughly $1 billion to implement seed and input interventions across twenty African countries between 2006 and 2020 (Wise, 2020). While the initiative promised to double yields and incomes for roughly 30 million smallholder farmers (which included many women) and cut SSA food insecurity rates in half, there is no documented evidence to date of AGRA's goals being met (Canfield, 2022; Wise, 2020). Nevertheless, the initiative had devastating consequences for African farmers by forcing them to incur debt cycles due to the high cost of required inputs like fertilizers and hybrid seeds, leading to dependence on monoculture practices—the same ones developed centuries prior during colonization that engendered similar environmental and health consequences.

Today, the corporate agricultural takeover in Africa is nearly complete, as multinational corporations such as Monsanto (now Bayer), Syngenta, and DuPont have monopolized the market on hybrid and genetically modified seeds, making African farmers reliant on global agribusiness for seeds and inputs (Hubbard, 2019). This "growth" has come at the expense of local farming communities and their motivations to preserve traditional farming techniques and suture ACB foodways. As Indian activist Vandana Shiva (2001) asserts in her book *Stolen Harvest: The Hijacking of the Global Food Supply*, "Over the past two decades every issue I have been engaged in as an ecological activist and organic intellectual has revealed that what the industrial economy calls 'growth' is really a form of theft from nature and people."

This industrial "growth" has also taken shape in different forms across parts of the Caribbean to further sever ACB foodways and local connections to land and food. In the USVI, arguably the biggest impact of the region's decision to shift from an agricultural-based economy to a tourism one has been the void it has left in local food environments—particularly among its low-income communities and communities-of-color (Gruver et al., 2024). While the islands have not experienced the same levels of overt neo-colonial takeover in recent years, such as the forced reliance on seed innovations and land theft and co-optation as African regions, the dearth of agriculture infrastructure has led to a quandary of increased dependence on cheap, unhealthy, and unsustainable food imports and simultaneous exporting of most locally grown food to global cash crop markets—leading to worsening rates of food insecurity and poor nutrition rates among Black Caribbeans (Barry et al., 2020).

These challenges have emerged against the backdrop of a shifting social and environmental landscape that has perpetuated the current on-the-ground realities. For example, as neoliberal development philosophies have materialized in recent years, they have infiltrated much of region's cultural psyche—where a focus on perceived social status, economic mobility, and the ability to adapt to Western cultural and consumption practices has supplanted traditional ways of life and food practices (Barry et al., 2020). When documenting the contemporary realities of the Caribbean food system, Tessa Barry and colleagues (2020) note:

> ...consuming imported foods, dining out at a multinational food chain, being able to regularly sip a Starbucks coffee, or passing through the nearest KFC for a daily snack box have all become just a few ways, either overt or even unwitting, to exhibit one's social rank and financial prowess. Hence, planting ground provisions at home in the yard versus procuring imported vegetables wrapped in plastic and polystyrene; or eating local fruits on the street/beach versus opting for Nestle sweets may not intentionally be ostentatious, but the historical trajectory of the Caribbean's food system, along with its agriculture sector, means these decisions are all as complex as they are political. (p. 107)

Paralleling this social shift are growing land ownership disparities in the region (Guannel et al., 2022). These trends have been accelerated, in part, due to a combination of interrelated economic phenomena, such as "climate gentrification" (a situation where increased climate risks, such as flooding or extreme weather, drive wealthy communities and developers to acquire land in safer and more climate-resilient areas—in the process displacing marginalized communities and exacerbating social and economic inequities) rising land values, discrepancies in heirs property and heritage rights, and a growing philanthropy and civic culture that privileges the economic interests and cultural values of the elite donor class (Bolin, 2024; James, 2020; Sarauw, 2024; Zhang & Mei, 2024). These conditions have made it almost impossible for Black

Caribbean farmers to politically and culturally influence the regional food system and preserve fractured foodways.

Today, this combined multitude of transgressions has created the current uneven landscape for global ACB communities in agriculture writ large. As such, inequities become embedded into the fabric of society, and they appear normal and commonsensical; it is usually at this stage that public health practitioners enter the conversation. Often guided by a well-intentioned nutrition or food access campaign and driven by public health values of beneficence, altruism, and equity, intervening at this point can be an exercise in futility in that programs get completely divorced from this important historical and structural context. In this way, relevant intervention efforts become similar to prescribing aspirin to alleviate pain associated with a pebble lodged in a shoe (e.g., short-term solutions, charity models, education campaigns), as opposed to removing the pebble altogether (e.g., redistributive land and agricultural justice policies). In today's neoliberal, "data-driven" public health landscape, these logics get normalized and reinforced via "resilience" discourses.

## Weathering the Storm: Resilience Policy in Public Health, Sustainability, and Agriculture

Against the backdrop of recent widespread social shocks such as COVID-19, racial injustice, and climate change, the concept of resilience has proliferated in public health and allied fields to draw the interest of both practitioners and researchers alike as a way for measuring how individuals and communities navigate responses to stress and adverse events. The American Psychological Association (n.d.) defines resilience as "the process of adapting in the face of adversity, trauma, tragedy, threats, or significant sources of stress," and includes things like disasters, racial discrimination, abuse, poverty, and witnessing violence. As the concept has gained popularity in public health specifically, several organizations and institutions have led the way in promulgating "resilience" philosophies into practice. For example, the National Association of County and City Health Officials (NACCHO) recently incorporated the "Building Community Resilience" framework as a best practice for addressing adverse childhood and community experiences among local health departments across the US in alignment with the tenets of Public Health 3.0 (Ellis & Dietz, 2017). The American Public Health Association, the flagship public health organization in the US, has sponsored trainings and led public conversations on the importance of communities to remain "resilient" in the face of adverse social shocks. Relatedly, the Centers for Disease Control and Prevention developed a Community Resilience Toolkit as a tool for assisting communities in their own resilience-building efforts (Pfefferbaum et al., 2013).

The concept of "resilience" is positioned in public health literature as particularly well-suited for studying ACB and other marginalized communities' responses to adverse events (Suslovic & Lett, 2024). A recent bevy of research articles and reports reflects a growing discourse in scientific and mainstream public health arenas (see Mushquash et al., 2021; Quinn et al., 2022; Taylor et al., 2022; Woods-Jaeger et al., 2020). Resilience discourses have also emerged in conversations on food systems (Hedberg, 2021). Considering that ACB and other underrepresented farmers and agriculturalists are particularly vulnerable to the myriad impacts of climate change (see Black, 2016; Dabone et al., 2021; Smith & Rhiney, 2016; Williams, 2021), agricultural experts and policymakers have sought ways to promote resiliency efforts among these groups. For example, a recent host of grant funding opportunities from institutions such as the National Institute of Food and Agriculture, Food and Agriculture Organization of the United Nations, and Climate Resilience Fund were made available to help build more "resilient" communities in the face of environmental and political shocks. Interdisciplinary agriculture and food researchers have built on this trend to explore resilience strategies of ACB and other marginalized communities (see Bowens, 2015; Jones, 2019; Quaicoe et al., 2024; Smolski & Schulman, 2024). Collectively, these trends have moved resilience from a popular buzzword to what Kate Derickson (2016) describes as "a normative civil good to which civil society groups and regional governments aspire" (p. 161).

Though resilience discourses have gained mainstream attention as a metaphor for envisioning sustainability and social change impacts in social science and public policy domains, the philosophy initially emerged out of the natural and physical sciences. Early definitions have foundational roots in physics and mathematics, where resilience is understood as "the capacity of a material or system to return to equilibrium after a displacement" (Norris et al., 2008, p. 127). Ecological scholars built upon this definition to include the concept of "ecological resilience," which goes beyond the mere capacity to withstand disturbances and underscores how ecosystems respond to external shocks by undergoing significant transformations—which can lead to the formation of new structures, behaviors, and patterns (Scordato & Gulbrandsen, 2024). As a framework for studying complex social phenomena (e.g., health disparities, resource distribution), ecological resilience is seen as more appropriate than earlier conceptions as it accounts for ongoing processes of adaptation, learning, and evolution (Stokols et al., 2013). Ecological resilience has grown to encompass other domains such as public policy, national security, public health, and urban planning (Mackinnon & Derickson, 2013).

## Interrogating Resilience

As resilience remains popular as an applicable framework for studying the processes of adaptation in response to adverse events, a growing number of scholarly critiques have emerged to highlight myriad shortcomings and challenges of the philosophy as a just and sustainable solution. A common criticism among this work suggests that ecological models of resilience work implicitly to reinforce the status quo by privileging established social structures, which are often shaped and upheld by unequal power relations (Evans, 2011; Hutcheon & Lashewicz, 2014; McDonnell, 2020). Previous scholarship has documented the ways that dominant public health resilience discourses focus on individual-level traits, often emphasizing biological and psychological aspects (e.g., coping, genetic resilience), while overlooking existing structural configurations that reify these conditions—leaving "vulnerable" communities on their own to develop resilience strategies (Chae et al., 2021; Shaw et al., 2016). Along these lines, scholars have interrogated how resilience discourses uphold racialized logics and capitalist economic structures (Grove et al., 2020; Suslovic & Lett, 2024). Given that capitalism conceals the racial and political nature of social systems, yet simultaneously "necessitates and produces racial difference" to sustain itself, critical work in this area draws parallels to how resilience discourses present as austere and politically neutral on the surface but obscure "the role of previous policies, institutions, and authorities in siphoning resources from poor neighborhoods of color in order to build resilience elsewhere" (Bonds, 2018, p. 1287).

Other critiques have explored how resilience governance functions as a largely technocratic endeavor where outside "experts" define problems and implement policies without engaging and/or incorporating the knowledge, skillsets, and capacities of local communities. In the context of agriculture and climate change, dominant resilience logics privilege "technical" approaches based on precision farming techniques, which favor scientific consensus and devalue farm heterogeneity—leaving little space for participatory approaches and localized knowledge (Darnhofer et al., 2016; Leach et al., 2012). Scholars in critical geography have explored the uneven ways resilience gets employed in social constructions of "place," arguing that the term is often inaccurate in terms of spatial scale, suggesting that its dominant logics position cities, regions, and local communities as autonomously functioning, self-organizing ecosystems that obscure their interconnections with broader structures (e.g., capital accumulation, state regulation; Davidson et al., 2016; Marston, 2000). Others in fields such as social work, behavioral science, and urban planning have highlighted how resilience discourses are constrained by hegemony, positivism, and ability-centrism (Coaffee & Rogers, 2008; Hutcheon & Lashewicz, 2014; Park et al., 2020).

Collectively, these scholarly interrogations highlight the expansive shortcomings and challenges of "resilience" as a prescriptive solution for marginalized communities to withstand adversarial events—requiring the need for more just and sustainable approaches. Following this corpus of criticisms, the next section introduces the politics of resourcefulness as the book's primary theoretical framework.

## Moving Beyond Resilience: Towards a Politics of Resourcefulness

In *Seeds of Sovereignty*, I employ *POR* as a guiding theoretical framework to document my ethnographic research process with the women of NWIAA to understand how they describe their lived experiences, political organizing strategies, and deep-rooted knowledge against the backdrop of intersectional inequity and structural violence. As a necessary corrective to dominant resilience philosophies, *POR* is a useful model for documenting and protecting ACB cultural assets and local knowledge and developing upstream community led-and-supported intervention models that animate more progressive and just social relations.

Mackinnon and Derickson (2013) describe *POR* as guided by four central axioms: resources, skill sets and technical knowledge, indigenous and "folk" knowledge, and recognition. *Resources* can be understood as a material and relational concept rather than an inherent community trait, and seek to interrogate the unequal distribution of resources by top-down structures that unduly impact low-income communities. Resources include things like organizing capacity, spare time, social capital, and also public and non-profit-sector investments. *Skill sets and technical knowledge* include things like community expertise in government procedures, financial matters, computing, and technology. *Indigenous and folk knowledge* offer alternative and collective ways of understanding the world, shaped by experiences, practices, and perceptions—what Escobar (2008) terms "alternative modernities." Such knowledge forms can provide critical "myths," or origin stories and explanatory frameworks, that combine dominant and observational insights to guide shared visions. Lastly, *recognition* fosters confidence, self-worth, and affirmation for individuals and communities, which can help mobilize existing resources and advocate for new ones. Recognition also grants group status based on shared social status and establishes the community as a rightful subject entitled to state resources and rights. While Mackinnon and Derickson (2013) describe recognition as something external in relation to local communities, I argue that recognition must also be identified internally by in-group stakeholders, which I explore in the subsequent empirical chapters. In the text, I apply *POR* axioms *resources*, *indigenous and "folk" knowledge*, and *recognition*.

*POR* has foundational roots in geography and wide application in sub-fields such as urban and city planning, climate change, and sustainability (Al-Humaiqani & Al-Ghamdi, 2023; Ranganathan & Bratman,

2021). More recently, the framework has been taken up by a wide range of scholars to study food systems transformation due to its applicability as a framework for critiquing resilience policy and activism. For example, Clare Clare Pettinger and colleagues (2024) applied resourcefulness to study food system inequities in the UK. Drawing on the community food researcher model "Food Systems Equality" (FoodSEqual) as a case study, the author's explored how such frameworks can facilitate food systems transformation by mobilizing local knowledge, facilitating relationship building (e.g., shared identities, support, reciprocity, and trust), community capacity building, and collaborative and co-productive approaches to research and stakeholder engagement. Anika Rice and colleagues (2023) applied resourcefulness to study pandemic-era economic shocks in Guatemala. Using data from eight *campesino* (i.e., small-scale farmers who use traditional farming methods) organizations, the author's highlighted how the participant's fostered resourcefulness through agroecology principles rooted in indigenous traditions, such as diversified farming practices, increased subsistence production, and reliance on community solidarity (e.g., informal local markets and barter systems). Relatedly, Chiara Tornaghi and Michiel Dehaene (2020) introduced resourcefulness as a form of urban political agroecology praxis, showcasing transformative food system practices in Riga, Rosario, Brussels, and London. Examples from their referenced case studies, such as "skills-land-exchange networks," urban agroecology coalitions, shared infrastructure development, and land justice initiatives, worked to challenge the systems and processes that shaped cities under capitalism.

*Seeds of Sovereignty* builds on this rich interdisciplinary work to highlight ACB women farmers' unique resourcefulness strategies as a case study for documenting combined bottom-up and grasstops political strategies and resource mobilization efforts and resisting dominant public health resilience logics.

# 3

# Forty Acres and a Lie

## Land Loss, a Cultural Backlash, and Interpersonal Challenges

"You hoop?"

"No, I used to. What about you?"

"Yeah, I could tell. Me? Nah, not anymore. I'm mostly focused on working with these kids right now."

THIS WAS PART OF MY conversation with Bridget Pettis, two-time Women's National Basketball Association (WNBA) champion, former assistant coach and executive, and NWIAA Arizona chapter leader, as we peeked in the basketball gym on the grounds of NWIAA's national headquarters building. Bridget is one of several chapter leaders who took up farming as a second career later in life after seeing the impact that growing food had on their local communities. Her passion for agriculture was initially sparked during her playing days in the WNBA, when she realized how the types of food she consumed affected her performance on the court. "That's something a professional athlete is very mindful about what we put in our body because we want to perform at our best. And that's what gave us our edge. So for me, it was [growing my own food]."

*Seeds of Sovereignty*. Andrew L. Carter, Oxford University Press. © Oxford University Press (2026).
DOI: 10.1093/9780197789391.003.0003

Despite a well-decorated career in basketball, she found that farming and agriculture allowed her to touch more people and impact her community in more poignant ways. “I didn’t realize my own self how important we are. I mean, we have the livelihood of our community right at our hands.... I see it as one of the most impactful positions in society today is a farmer. Way more impactful than a basketball player!” In 2020, Bridget left her position as assistant coach of the WNBA’s Chicago Sky to take on a new career trajectory and follow her passion for farming. Today, she runs Project Roots, a non-profit organization that provides locally grown food to underserved communities in Phoenix, Arizona.

Back at NWIAA headquarters, after mimicking turnaround jump shots and post moves on the empty court, Bridget and I rejoined the group of a dozen or so individuals getting a tour of the facility. Bridget and I were part of over 100 people present for the National Women in Agriculture Association’s fifteenth year anniversary conference and farm expo on February 21–22, 2023. The two-day event, which took place at the Meinders School of Business at Oklahoma City University (a private institution located just up the road in northern Oklahoma City) and NWIAA’s headquarters building, was meant to celebrate the organization’s quindecennial year in existence and bring together chapter leaders from its seventy-plus locations in the United States, the US Virgin Islands, and Africa. Representatives from various Department of Agriculture offices, including the National Resource Conservation Service and Farm Service Agency, among other private and public vendors were on hand to pass out brochures and offer free advice and counsel to the conferencegoers in attendance (see Figure 3.1). The event saw a wide variety of guest speakers and panel presentations, including a panel of retired professional athletes from the National Basketball Association, National Football League, and WNBA, who started second careers as entrepreneurs in agriculture, officers from the United States Department of Agriculture (USDA) Foreign Agriculture Services and the United States Agency for International Development, and remarks from Oklahoma state legislators, US Congresspeople, and members of the House Committee on Agriculture (see Figure 3.2). The event culminated with a chapter leader roll call (where each chapter leader introduced themselves, which region they represented, and provided

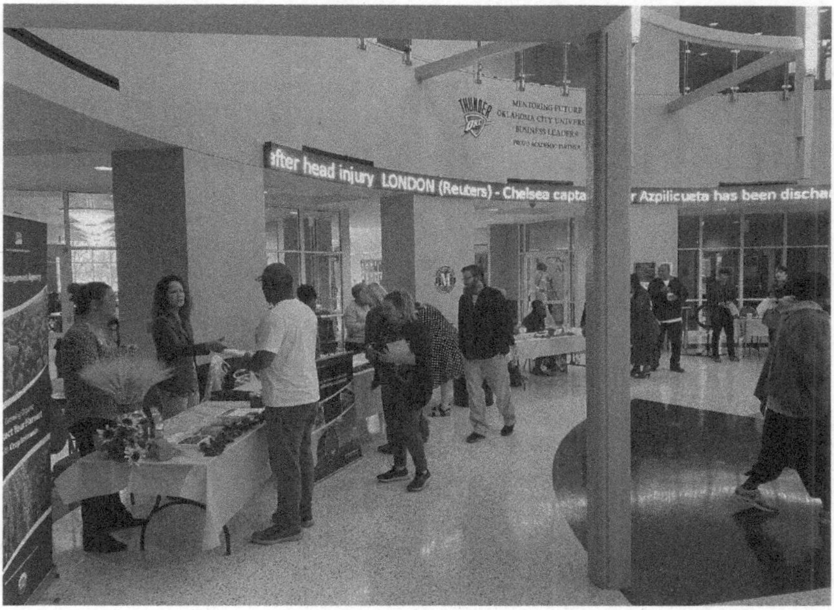
after head injury LONDON (Reuters) - Chelsea capta
r Azpilicueta has been discha

**FIGURE 3.1** Vendors speak with attendees at the agriculture resource fair during NWIAA's fifteenth-year anniversary conference on February 21, 2023.

Photo by author

general chapter updates) and farm expo (where participants boarded buses to tour local farms in the Oklahoma City area). For attendees, NWIAA's fifteenth anniversary was more than just an opportunity to engage in fellowship and celebration but symbolized a form of resistance that fostered a dialogic space to develop alternative agendas and challenge existing power relations in agriculture by building organizing capacity, social capital, and capturing public and third sector resources.

The rhetorical situation[1] that birthed NWIAA's fifteenth-year anniversary conference does not exist in a vacuum and is situated within a

[1] A "rhetorical situation," as defined by American rhetorician Lloyd Bitzer, is the context in which communication takes place, where a speaker is prompted to respond to an exigence (i.e., crisis) through persuasive discourse, addressing an audience capable of influencing change, and navigating constraints that shape the response. It emphasizes the interaction between the situation, speaker, and audience in shaping effective rhetoric.

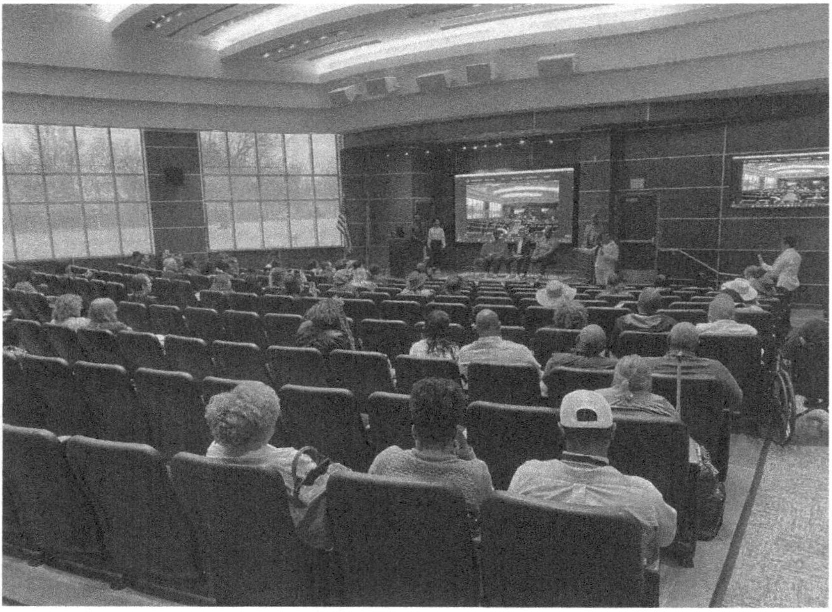

**FIGURE 3.2** Professional athletes in agriculture panel at NWIAA's fifteenth-year anniversary conference on February 21, 2023.

Photo by author

social context rife with pervasive forms of racial and gendered capitalism, which work to support "divide and conquer" philosophies across divisions of labor and disband cultural groups and assets, cultural cooptation and erasure, and legacies of settler colonialism. In this chapter, I bring together some of this broader context to paint the current political conditions for ACB women farmers. This chapter is broken down into two main sections. The first section opens with an oral history account of NWIAA executive director and founder Tammy Gray-Steele and her family's unique history and entry point into agriculture. The brief account underscores some of the current challenges ACB farmers face and provokes Black futurist imaginings of land ownership and community sovereignty given different social and political circumstances. After this context is detailed, the second section of the chapter provides an ethnographic window into the diverse relational barriers the women of NWIAA experienced when navigating dominant agricultural spaces. While subsequent chapters in the book will document the women's lived narratives against the backdrop of broader structural contexts, drawing specific attention to how they discuss on-the-ground interpersonal encumbrances is important to document because these more direct, micro-forms of inequity often emerge *after* communities gain access to dominant cultural spaces and resources—a necessary (but oft undertheorized) step interventionists describe for achieving equity. The intersectional analysis provides a study-specific context to the historical narrative detailed in the previous chapter.

## From Dispossession to Disenfranchisement: Situating the Sociopolitical Battlefield That Birthed the Fight for ACB Agricultural Justice

My academic community partnership with the women of NWIAA was forged in September 2021 during the height of the COVID-19 pandemic. At the time, I was interviewing Black farmers across the United States to learn more about their self-described challenges and unique opportunities in agriculture during the pandemic as a part of my broader decade-long research agenda centering Black farmer culture and knowledge preservation, community food security, structural discrimination, and political and economic mobilization narratives. Through a serendipitous social connection with one of my academic colleagues at the University of Oklahoma, I was introduced to Alaric, a Black farmer in Northeast Oklahoma who ran a farm incubator program that used vertical farming and hydroponics to support local food security efforts and promote community empowerment. During our discussion, he reflected on the many challenges Black farmers experience today and how many of those same challenges persisted in the decades prior.

> So I did some [social media] posts this morning, just doing research and just looking at kind of the history of Black farmers. Back in '86, I mean, you had reports by the Washington Post that talks about the decline of Black farmers in 1986. And here it is 2021, going into '22, and they're still writing those same articles. So most of the farming that I've seen, especially out here in Oklahoma and other states, is something that's been passed down. But the problem is that there

> becomes a point where there's nobody to pass it down to because [Black farmers], as they grow up, haven't made farming continue to be something that's economic, that makes the next generation want to get involved, that there's a lucrative business there for me to get involved with.

Alaric's point about replacing the aging and rapidly declining Black farming population was nothing new—there have been an abundance of research papers, newspaper articles, and critical think pieces dedicated to this exact topic over the past several decades, and it has gained increasingly more attention across mainstream media outlets (Bustillo, 2023; Gugliotta, 1990; Reynolds, 2002). However, his comments piqued my interest to learn more about what was happening on the ground specifically in Oklahoma. Luckily for me, Alaric's strong connection within the local Black farming community led me to other Oklahoman farmers, including NWIAA's executive director, Tammy Gray-Steele, whose story would profoundly impact the trajectory of my research.

When Tammy and I first met, I was immediately enthralled by her unique background and lived experiences. We talked for over two hours during our first conversation, where she went into great detail about her origin story as a Black woman farmer in the United States, sharing poignant narratives about the unique intersectional barriers and mobilizing triumphs women like her endured. In true journalistic fashion, I tried my best to jot down and capture as many powerful vignettes as I could as she remarked rapid-fire memories in 10–15-minute soundbites. Inspired by her narrative, I reached out again a few days after our call with interest in documenting a more comprehensive account of ACB women and NWIAA—laying the early foundations for this manuscript.

The more Tammy shared with me about how she got into agriculture, I learned about her family's unique farming history and became interested in how their experience could provide a case study for exploring the trajectory of Black farmers in the United States writ large and the "broken promise" that could have reshaped the current national and global agriculture and food economy. Dating back to 1913, Tammy's great-grandparents were recipients of the elusive "40 acres" mandate promised to Black freedmen as a part of Special Field Orders #15 after the Civil War (see Figure 3.3). In places like Oklahoma, many members of the Five Tribes (Cherokee, Chickasaw, Choctaw, Muscogee, Seminole) owned slaves before the war, but were mandated by the US government to accept them as tribal members (classified as "Freedman") as a part of the Dawes Severalty Act during Reconstruction. Further, the Tribes were forced to divide their communally owned land into private individual allotments to encourage their assimilation into mainstream society and promote capitalist investment by non-Indians (Roberts, 2021). During land redistribution efforts, Black Oklahoman tribal members received more allotments in comparison to Freedmen

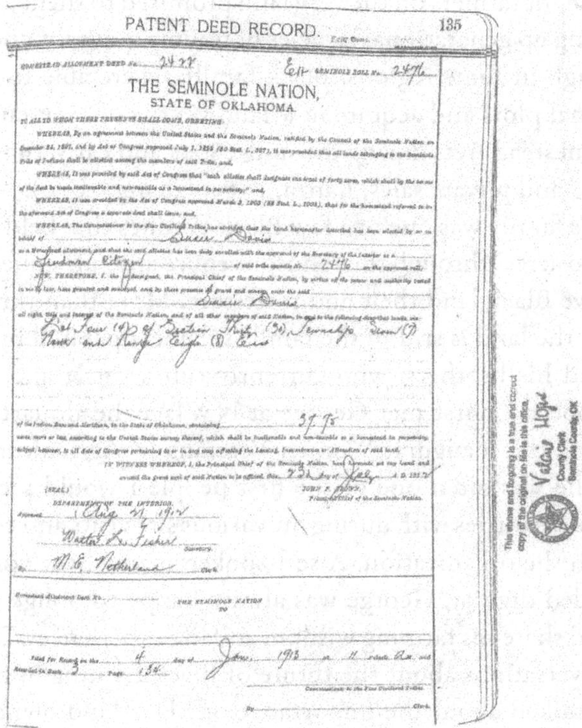


**FIGURE 3.3** Tammy's Grandparents' Homestead Allotment "40 acres" deed issued by the Seminole Nation of Oklahoma on January 4, 1913.
Photo by Tammy Gray-Steele

living in other parts of the South. For example, in the Muscogee Nation, almost one-third of the land was owned by Black Freedmen, who were among the fastest tribal members to register for allotments when they became available, receiving much of the prime farmland in the region (Helfrich et al., 2021).

However, as documented in the previous chapter, the promise was quickly reversed as Andrew Johnson reversed the mandate as soon as he entered office following Abraham Lincoln's assassination. Johnson's rich legacy of racist governance, including the enactment of the Black Codes post-Civil War and opposition to the Freedman Bureau's would further disenfranchise Black Freedmen. Without land of their own to farm, many Freedmen were left with no choice but to work as sharecroppers and tenant farmers on the very land promised to them just months prior, setting up generational legacies of trauma, poverty, and financial debt (though in some regions, Black families were able to hold onto their original plots and acquire new land via the uneven enforcement of the Homestead Acts during the mid-1800s and early 1900s, various "land runs," and private sales; Lanza, 1999; Chang, 2010).

Tammy's family was one of a few Black families that held onto their original "40 acres" through the Johnson tenure and subsequent decades of collective Black land theft and forfeiture. More than three generations later, the land is still in the family's name, operated by her uncle George and his brothers, who currently run a cattle and goat farm on the property. I first met George at NWIAA headquarters in July 2022 during the inaugural Women Veterans in Agriculture Conference, and he was often one of the first people I would seek out and exchange pleasantries with during my various site visits and community events with the organization. A soft-spoken man whose voice carried an embedded dignity, George was always happy to oblige me in discussion and share his farming wisdom and life experiences. During one of our conversations about the future of Black farming in the United States, he talked about the importance of Black land ownership and the consistent challenges he faced trying to maintain his family's land.

> It's been challenging trying to maintain [our land] all of these years and keep everybody focused and trying to keep them to understand the history—I call it generational wealth is what they was leaving us,

> even though they probably weren't aware of it at the time because that's something they don't make anymore is land. And so they could have left us a million dollars and it would have been gone by now, 112 years. So the land is still there and the house is 100 years old and it's still there.

Like other Black families who own land, the consistent threat of forfeiture via lack of understanding its long-term value, discrimination and exploitation, predatory practices such as heirs' property laws,[2] and outright violence and theft, has remained a source of concern for George and his brothers (see Figures 3.4 and 3.5). Characterizing inherited land as a form of "generational wealth" is not a relatable metaphor among much of the Black community today—Black land ownership in the United States has diminished by 90 percent during the twentieth century, equating to over $326 billion in collective land loss (Francis et al., 2022). Growing up in a multigenerational home, George witnessed these disturbing trends unfold in real time. He reflected during one of our conversations on the dramatic shift in land ownership in his local community over the years. "In the neighborhood that we live in, it used to be all Blacks, now we are the only Blacks that live there... We are the fly in the buttermilk out here."

George's self-perception as a "fly in the buttermilk" is a historical trope that draws on DuBoisian connotations of double consciousness in "always looking at oneself through the eyes" of the dominant group; the idiom is commonly used to symbolize the experience of being marked materially and discursively "Other" and an unwelcome presence (Scott, 2009). James Baldwin famously coined "fly in the buttermilk" as a metaphor in his eponymously titled essay to describe the experiences of Black students integrating into predominantly white schools during the Civil Rights Movement in the 1960s. The essay

---

[2] Heirs' property is land passed down through generations without a formal will, resulting in shared ownership among multiple heirs. This often leads to unclear property titles, with ownership split among family members, making it difficult to sell or maintain the land. Heirs' property laws have disproportionately impacted Black families in the United States, contributing to widespread land loss as fragmented ownership which enables exploitation, forced sales, and legal challenges, ultimately eroding generational wealth.

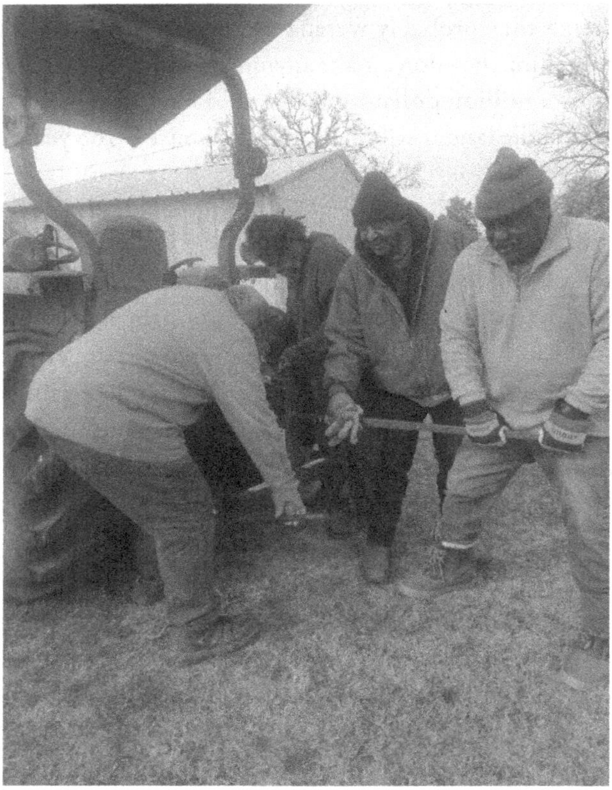

FIGURE 3.4 George and his brothers working on a tractor on their family farm in Wewoka, Oklahoma.

Photo by Tammy Gray-Steele

painted a vivid picture of isolation and marginalization among the students and their consistent need to demonstrate validity and worthiness to their white peers and teachers. Similarly, in the context of agriculture, George described experiences of trying to remain relevant and taken seriously in dominant spaces by white farmers that did not want him there—referencing multiple examples of overt and inferential acts of discrimination. With a shaky tremble in his voice to hide his frustration, he recounted one particular incident during the 1980s where he suspected that white farmers burned his farmhouse down and he was unable to use insurance money to rebuild the home, subsequently leading to diminished property values.

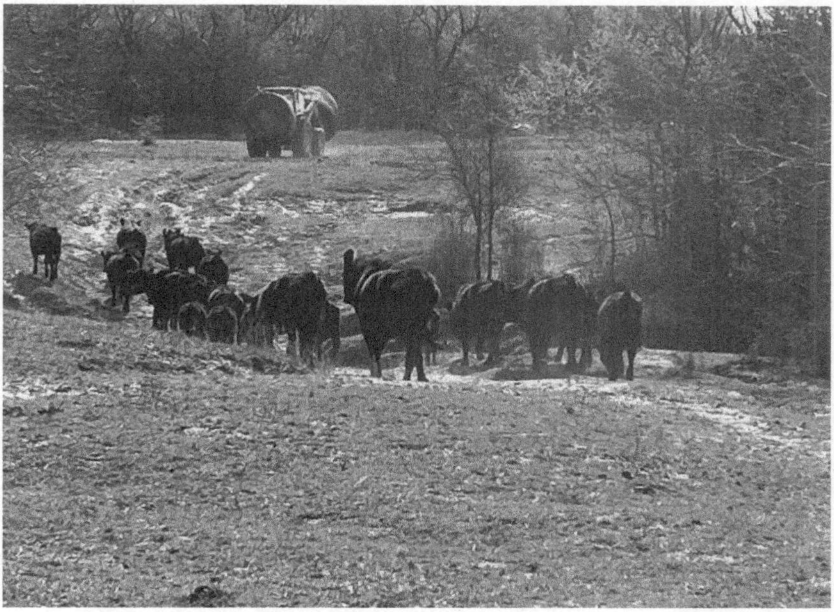

**FIGURE 3.5** A herd of cattle at George's family farm.
Photo by Tammy Gray-Steele

> I had a three-bedroom home on my 80-acre site that I was fortunate to get financed. Okay. Well, like I was telling you, we're the only Blacks out here. And Whites don't really care for us that much, but I feel like I couldn't prove it, but I feel like they're the one that destroyed my home because it was burned down. And so instead of USDA letting me use the insurance money to rebuild, I was behind on my loans. So they said, 'No, you had to pay the loan. Take the insurance money and pay it towards the loan.' I thought that was a part of discrimination, because of that my land is going to go down in value because there's no house on it. And I felt like [the USDA] should have let me use the money to rebuild my house. So that way, the value of the property would have stayed up because if you ain't got no home on it, all you got is raw land.

Without substantiated evidence to prove otherwise, George remained resolute in his belief that the incident was an example of overt racial violence and representative of some of the same political red tape the USDA historically wielded to hold back Black farmers. In addition to experiencing direct forms of hatred and violence, George also talked about the level of daily, micro-level insults Black farmers experience that accumulate over time and in some ways are more impactful in dispiriting their motivations and mobilizing efforts, such as having to prove their competence and agriculture expertise and prohibitive legalese in the farm-loan process, making it difficult to remain sustainable and pass down generational land and farms to younger generations. Strapped with these burdensome challenges, George and his brothers have not only survived, but *thrived* in the agriculture industry, despite their "fly in the buttermilk" status; in recent decades, they pooled their resources and secured additional plots of land on adjacent properties, expanding the family's original 40-acre allotment into what is now 800-plus acres. Yet, despite these successes, George and his brothers find themselves in a constant state of precarity, as public support for Black farmers wanes depending on which presidential administration is in office and the social climate of a given era. Today, he remains cautiously optimistic for the continued momentum generated by the renewed public interest in Black farmer struggles.

> I just pray that—the different presidents get in and it's not thrown to the back burner again. I don't know who's the right one to help this type of thing, but you would think that everybody should be encouraged to help youngsters, future generations on the way our country is going to grow.

Today, the undergirding tenacity and perseverance of George and Tammy's family's "40 acres and a mule" account is popular folklore among Oklahomans and has received significant national spotlight. Locally, news outlets regularly write human interest segments about their resilience as Black farmers, while national news outlets such as CBS and NBC feature the family's story as an entry point into bigger conversations about the current state of Black farmers (Moss, 2023). The Steele family farm was given a dedicated segment on cultural critic W. Kamau Bell's popular CNN television series *United Shades of America* in 2020 (see Figure 3.6).

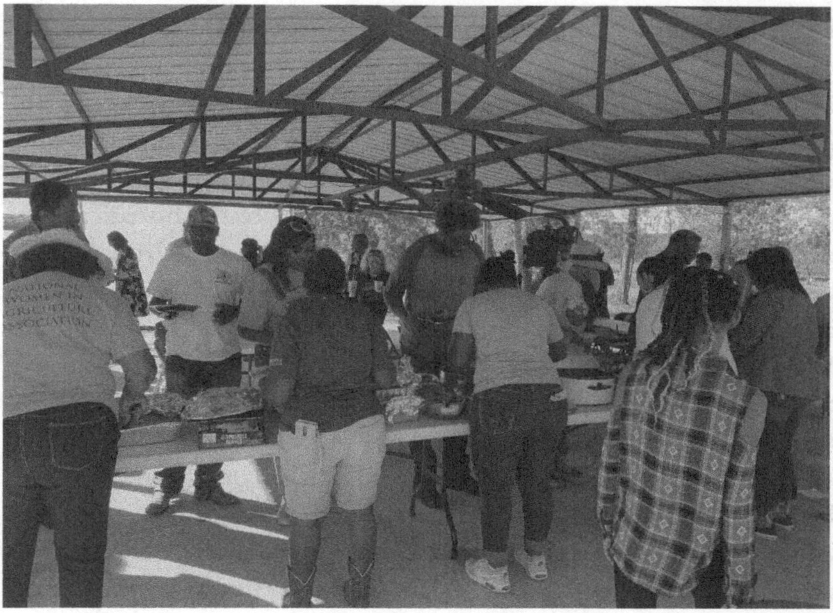

**FIGURE 3.6** A behind-the-scenes photo of Tammy, W. Kamau Bell, and members of her extended family at the family farm, taken during the filming of *United Shades of America.*

Photo by Tammy Gray-Steele

As a synecdoche for racial progress, this inspiring familial history represents more than a romanticized agrarian notion of resilience and family values, but sheds light on how a strategically devised and long-term land reform initiative might have impacted current on-the-ground Black wealth and health disparities in the United States and globally. For example, had the original "40 acres" mandate been upheld and protected throughout history, several experts have estimated that the collective wealth of Black communities nationally would be valued at ***$6.4 trillion today*** (Kawachi, 2022). Given the fact that the majority of wealth in the United States comes from inheritance and in vivo cash transfers, the deprivation of land ownership and wealth among the Black community has had dramatic intergenerational effects (Darity Jr. & Nicholson, 2005).

Against the backdrop of the 2020 social crises, a bevy of interdisciplinary scholars reopened past conversations about the potential of large-scale social reforms, such as land redistribution initiatives and reparations, to address the longstanding social, health, and economic inequities among Black communities in the United States. In the public health realm, myriad research articles, reports, and presentations have proliferated across leading academic institutions, popular press outlets, and government agencies to situate the historical context and provide potential praxis-oriented solutions. Critical think pieces from the New England Journal of Medicine ("Reparations as a Public Health Priority—A Strategy for Ending Black-White Health Disparities"), Harvard T. H. Chan School of Public Health ("Perspective: How Black Reparations Could End Health Disparities"), and Columbia University Mailman School of Public Health ("A Public Health Case for Reparations") were published in the months following George Floyd's death to bring public attention to the topic. Aligning with this mainstream consciousness shift, US Congress introduced HR 40 in 2021, which established the Commission to Study and Develop Reparation Proposals for African Americans to "examine slavery and discrimination in the colonies and the United States from 1619 to the present and recommend appropriate remedies" (Congress.gov, 2021). Some primary tasks of the Commission were to identify:

(1) the role of the federal and state governments in supporting the institution of slavery,
(2) forms of discrimination in the public and private sectors against freed slaves and their descendants, and
(3) lingering negative effects of slavery on living African Americans and society.

Relatedly, in California, state leadership developed the first Reparations Task Force, a governor-appointed body to study and develop proposals for African American reparations in 2020. The Task Force explored areas such as housing discrimination, education, healthcare, and carceral system inequities from the state's founding in 1850 to today (Lewis et al., 2023). In 2023, the Task Force released a preliminary report to provide "incontrovertible evidence of the harms requiring reparations and meaningful recommendations designed to redress them," with final policy proposals scheduled to come in the months following (Lewis et al., 2023, p. 2).

On the surface, the social moment had all the ingredients necessary to spearhead a sustainable and widespread transformative justice movement to a degree never seen before in US history. However, like many other promising initiatives that emerged during the 2020 period of racial reckoning, many of these initiatives have lost their momentum. Today, an equal and opposite backlash—or "whitelash," as author Wesley Lowery (2023) puts it—has emerged to challenge these progresses. This pushback has taken multifarious forms, including President Trump's nomination of a historically conservative Supreme Court, widespread resistance to popular social movements and initiatives such as Black Lives Matter and Defund the Police, anti-DEI policies in higher education, regressive laws around gender and sexual orientation, the emergence of new Right-wing and religious nationalist movements such as Project 2025, among others (Borg, 2024; McGregor & Rosenberg, 2020; Ebbinghaus et al., 2024).

In the context of agriculture, this "whitelash," undergirded by racial capitalism logics, has also surfaced at a fervent level to quell any meaningful equitable policy legislation discussions. Examples such as the Emergency Relief for Farmers of Color Act (ERFCA) repeal and the uneven funding of the Climate-Smart Commodities initiative have largely upheld existing inequities in the sector. Other ambitious efforts, such as HR 40 and the California reparations bill, were also heavily modified or abrogated in subsequent months[3] (Holden, 2024). This cumulative loss of momentum has positioned Black farmers in a familiar situation—left to fend for themselves to self-mobilize resources and levy political support. For ACB women farmers, these retributive actions cut even deeper as they are situated against embedded histories of intersectional race and gender inequities. This is the sociopolitical battlefield in which the women of NWIAA found themselves...

[3] Despite its transformative potential, the reparations proposals were ultimately blocked by California's Legislative Black Caucus on August 31, 2024. The move was largely a result of combined concerns about the long-term financial commitment needed to develop the required infrastructure, political and public resistance, and strategic disagreements among the Caucus itself between creating more immediate, concrete steps prior to instituting the bill (Fry et al., 2024; Zavala, 2024).

## Overlooked and Underestimated: Exploring the Relational Barriers of ACB Women to Agriculture

After I established my partnership with NWIAA, I immediately got to work doing formative research to learn more about the organization and the individual stories of its chapter leaders and members. Some of these early activities consisted of perusing the chapter leaders' affiliated webpages and other publicly available information, attending their various workshops and networking events, and setting up interviews to learn more about who they were as farmers and their motivations for wanting to be a part of a women's advocacy collective. From my early investigations, the rife transformative power embedded in their stories was palpable. During a roll call at a training workshop I attended, I remarked on the sheer diversity of cultural and social identities of the women in attendance, which spanned multiple generations and diverse global regions. From a public health lens, the connections the women made to food security and broader structural and ideological influences were both inherent and transparent. I immediately began asking *who were these women doing this impactful work without a platform or political support?* And *why weren't they being talked about in mainstream contexts, particularly in the current social climate of advocating for diverse voices and identities in positions of power?*

The concept was not just lost on me. For example, when I would tell people about my work with these women at academic conferences and other professional settings, the reactions ranged from general interest and curiosity ("wow, that's so cool!") to variations of bewilderment and incredulousness ("wait, [Black women farmers] are really a thing?"). As noted in the previous chapters, popular discourses have deemed Black women farmers fundamentally obsolete—a faceless, combined mere 1 percent of both Black and women farmers (USDANASS, 2017b). In the United States, examples such as the USDA segmenting resources by lumping Black women into the nebulous "socially disadvantaged farmers" category and the lack of representation in leadership among Black agrarian communities have largely erased Black women farmers' voice and political agency in dominant agriculture and public health platforms. Similar trends have emerged in African and Caribbean contexts, as women consistently struggle to own and operate land and receive support from their local and national governments (Barry & Gahman, 2021; Brixiová et al., 2020; Slavchevska et al., 2021). These realities were not lost on the participants, as they embodied these scars of injustice as they went about their day-to-day lives. Many of the women described how their mere physical presence, cultural practices, and self-assurance as agricultural experts challenged hegemonic norms in the agricultural spaces they frequented, often resulting in them experiencing relational forms of micro- and macro-aggressive insults and limiting their capacity to access resources, build social networks, be seen as reputable, and politically mobilize to address community food security issues.

For Diana (USVI chapter leader), a farmer of Black Caribbean ancestry who lived most of her adult life split between South Florida and St. Croix, the United States Virgin Islands, gaining legitimacy in agricultural leadership roles was a persistent challenge she had to overcome throughout her life. Her drive for farming education and youth development was first instilled by her grandfather, who would regularly explain complex agricultural principles to her without having traditional training. "He didn't have a formal education, but he was the most educated person I knew because he read a lot and he had a thirst for knowledge...and as an agriculturist, he was applying scientific techniques, not recognizing the impact." As a Black Caribbean growing up in Trinidad, her grandfather faced immense discrimination and was denied opportunities to enter higher education. After learning more about his personal experiences, Diana became galvanized to pursue some of the same educational opportunities previously denied to him. "He encouraged me to pursue higher education. And I promised him that I would do formally what he couldn't do formally." As she went on to pursue her tertiary education while enrolled as an undergraduate student in an agriculture degree program at the University of Florida, she was brought into intimately uncomfortable contact with the same landscape of racial discrimination that burdened her grandfather across the Caribbean and has historically marked farm education programs in the United States and globally.

> I studied at University of Florida. I am Caribbean. I am Black. I have dreadlocks. I have an accent. I went into agriculture at University of Florida beginning in the '80s. I used to go as a summer student here.

> I had a degree here in agriculture but they didn't do art education. I had an associate degree. So they gave me a chance to teach middle school when I was 19. And then in the summers, I would travel to US, pay out of state fees, stay on their campus and take six credits in low education type course just to do that. And the level of disregard—I can't even call it discrimination. The level of disregard by other students and faculty, the level of discomfort they had for me being so different from what they were used to, that discomfort. Those things showed me the bias there was in agriculture.

While Diana did not experience the same levels of overt discrimination as her grandfather, such as being outright denied opportunities to pursue higher education, her program's faculty and students "disregard" for her viewpoints and feelings of discomfort was equally impactful on her self-concept and affirmed the broader cultural hegemony in agriculture education. Even as she moved ahead in her career to assume leadership positions, such as a high school agriculture teacher, she still had to navigate racist and sexist indignities by her white students who didn't take her seriously as a Black Caribbean woman:

> I taught agriculture at South Dade High School in Homestead, that's the southernmost FFA [Future Farmers of America] chapter in the nation. When I started teaching there, all my students were redneck students. They never had a female teacher, and they never had a Black teacher, and they got me. And with me, I [told them] they can discriminate against me, my look, my accent, my race, my everything else, but excellence they can't discriminate against. So that has always been my mantra. Anything I do, I do with excellence. So even if they don't like you, everybody wants to be on the team that's winning, somebody who has been far.

Diana described another time when she was asked by her school's administration to find ways to make their agriculture program (which at the time was made up of predominantly rural white students) more representative of the school population (located in South Florida). She noticed that when she started bringing in non-white students from Haitian, Mexican, and Black backgrounds to participate in farm education activities, her white students were inclined to assume leadership roles and assign others traditionally labor-intensive and low-prestige tasks, such as picking beans and weeding, while they assigned themselves higher-prestige positions such as driving tractors. Backed into an uncomfortable position, rather than complain or quit her position, Diana took on the challenge of changing her white students' mindset, describing the situation as a "cultural racial experiment."

Diana's experiences highlight the additional unforeseen barriers ACB women experience as they take on leadership and expert-level positions. As Diana moved ahead into more influential positions of leadership, rather than being seen as building on the descriptive and intellectual diversity of her school, she was isolated and still not taken seriously by her white colleagues and students, having to prove her worth and capacity to them. Her dissonance between feeling responsible for changing the racist attitudes of her students but not wanting to challenge existing structures builds on the politics of performance legacies that are often imposed on Black Caribbean women like her in leadership positions. Caribbean scholar Cecilia Green (2006) has explored the origins of Afro-Caribbean women's imposed racial, gendered, and sexual status, examining the cultural and structural conditions that create a contradictory legacy of constraint and autonomy. Green highlights how a combination of Eurocentric middle-class "respectability" and Afrocentric subaltern "self-respect" has shaped the economic and occupational spaces these women are forced to navigate. In the context of agriculture, this legacy has created additional barriers for Caribbean women to fully express personal agency in dominant social and professional settings.

In addition to barriers in agricultural education leadership contexts, many of the women talked about not being taken seriously for their expertise and mobilizing potential by other farmers. Juhna (US Missouri chapter leader), a self-described city girl from Chicago, was not exposed to agriculture growing up and became interested after experimenting with a backyard garden as an adult. Through her explorations, her passion quickly grew after she purchased a small plot of land to start growing food for her local community. However, as her business grew larger and she started entering mainstream agricultural spaces, her expertise was constantly questioned, and she was not given the benefit of the doubt as a Black woman farmer and constantly had to push back against harmful stereotypes of Black communities around food and agriculture. She reflected on a time when she assumed not to possess a serious interest in farming by her internship preceptor simply because she was a Black woman.

> Actually, I interned for a farm that a white couple owned. And when I got to telling them because I had already studied plant migration. I'm in a master's gardener class. When I started studying, I'm already good enough. When I start, they start talking to me as if I didn't know. See, and that's another thing we get. We get people who talk to you as if you're incompetent. 'Baby steps. Oh, you like—would you like daisies, flowers?' No, I'm not doing no flowers. I'm doing production. I'm doing food. I'm doing sustainable things that can sustain me, self-sustain myself. And when I started telling them all the things, they were surprised because they didn't even think that I researched. They don't think that myself as a Black woman or as a minority, that would have enough sense or enough skill to research what they're talking about, to research the laws, to research the policies, to research for the time of the day.

Nearly all of the women echoed a similar version of Juhna's story being overlooked for their expertise and serious interest in farming by other farmers, who chose to focus on ACB women's limited numbers and marginalization status, rather than highlight their unique assets, such as their community-building potential, inherent agricultural skillsets, and innovative approaches toward addressing community food security.

The social and political backdrop that undergirded the participants' experiences generated additional "double barriers" they had to navigate. For instance, their cultural erasure and limited representation in agriculture granted them low political agency across political and ideological battlefields on the one hand; simultaneously, the global political moment spearheaded by the murder of George Floyd and 2020 social crises created a grant-funding environment in the public and private sectors where increased money were allocated for social responsibility campaigns that incorporated the "participation" of underrepresented groups in the development of top-down "innovation" projects—leaving their stories and agricultural experiences rife for theft and co-optation (Hing et al., 2024; Jan et al., 2021; Lett et al., 2022). Vivian (US

Tennessee chapter leader), a lifelong agriculturalist in her own right and one of NWIAA's eldest stateswomen and official chaplain, identified this precarious position of marginality after spending years in Washington D.C. advocating for Black women farmer rights. During one of our conversations, I asked her why she felt policymakers and USDA officials did not take Black women's advocacy efforts seriously, to which she bluntly replied, "Because we're women. People don't want to listen to us—they want to hear us, but they're not listening to us. They're not taking us serious about what we want to do."

Vivian's conviction of wanting to be *heard* but not *listened to* by policymakers and other agricultural leadership is reflective of some of the same performative allyship rhetorics that Kutlaca & Radke (2023) describe as "easy and costless actions that often do not challenge the status quo and are motivated primarily by the desire to accrue personal benefits" (p. 1). Alexis (US Georgia chapter member), a hemp and cannabis farmer whose father was the first Black hemp lobbyist in the state of Georgia, similarly experienced feelings of being *heard* but not *listened to*, detailing examples of being surveilled and co-opted for her agricultural knowledge by top-down power brokers in agriculture—such as ACB women's cultural capital and expertise being extracted via community "listening sessions" under the guise of participation and community buy-in and forcing them to take aptitude tests to assess their worthiness for receiving help.

> I would say [the USDA is] parasitic . . . because, like I said, a lot of times as Black women, you have to write an essay or prove your worthiness when, in fact, they came to you. You see what I mean? They came into our community because your work is so good, and we want to know what you're doing, how you're doing it, but then treat you like you don't have value or you're not smart enough to realize [the USDA] is taking this same information, making programs, and then bringing it back to the community and saying, 'Would you like a job from us from all the information we took from you and then made a program for?' That's parasitic versus saying, 'Oh, I see you have a business,' or, 'Maybe we can start business incubators with you to promote positioning you for the bank loan to get land acquisition,' you see what I mean? Versus what they usually do. It's like, okay, well, we can do technical assistance meetings all day, and nobody's really getting anything done.

Alexis's interpretation of such community engagement strategies as "parasitic" aligns with similar critiques made by interdisciplinary public health and development communication scholars who have highlighted the ways in which development models work to co-opt resources, knowledge forms, and authority from deficit-framed "targeted" communities (Alkon & Cadji, 2020; Millar, 2018). In the context of public health, extractive actions such as the ones described by Alexis work to obscure how disparities in food security and access begin and are maintained at the food production level by limiting the innovation of nondominant actors and alternative knowledge, such as ACB women farmers' historical lived experiences, political voice, and shared deep-rooted agricultural expertise to address such inequities.

The women's mere physical presence and social identity marked their bodies and cultural practices as non-normative in the spaces they frequented, forcing them to either assimilate to traditional conventions or be characterized as indignant rabble-rousers. In situations where the participants asserted their agricultural expertise and attempted to "take up" space when engaging with top-down gatekeepers, they were overcome with double consciousness and were keenly attuned to how their positionality could be viewed as a threat or offensive. Juhna (US Missouri chapter leader) and Selena (US North Carolina chapter leader), a blueberry farmer and floriculturist, reflected on how they internalized these experiences.

> Who's going to give you a chance? They put you down. What they do is they try to deter you because they're scared. When you're not scared, and you're here to push the envelope, they're scared.
>
> *(JUHNA)*

> Oftentimes, I think people feel—sometimes, we can feel intimidated when you're a strong Black woman or educated Black woman. And there's really no need to be. So it stops the work or pauses the work because even the people that may be in power are intimidated. And so if you have to go to someone to sign a check and they're intimidated by you, it's harder to get the check signed.
>
> *(SELENA)*

The women also described how they found themselves pitted against men in relational contexts, which forced them to navigate dynamic, embedded white heteronormativity present in dominant agricultural spaces and rooted patriarchy in Black agrarianism and leadership spaces in their quest to secure resources and political power, spanning ACB contexts (Tyler, 2020). Jadae (US New Jersey chapter leader), a cattle and livestock farmer who got into agriculture through homesteading after her mother was diagnosed with an autoimmune condition, and Keturah (Virgin Islands Women in Agriculture Association chapter member), a new farmer whose passion for growing food was first cultivated during her undergraduate campaign at the University of Virgin Islands School of Agriculture, talked about how intersectional barriers manifested relationally during their interactions with men in leadership positions:

> One of the difficulties as a female farmer has been it is a good old boys' game. They do not want to impart wisdom. They do not want to impart resources. They do not want to collaborate on anything... And as for race, like I said, without being grandfathered in or generational farming, most Black people do not have the funds to start farming. Me and my mother started our family farm, and we both work two jobs. We do not have farmhands. We do not have employees.
>
> *(JADAE)*

> The only challenge I would say is other farmers not having faith in your work ethic, just not believing that you're strong enough, not believing that you could do the work that their other man workers are doing. That's the only challenge that I've experienced, and just them not taking you seriously as a farmer.
>
> *(KETURAH)*

In Africa, relational race barriers were not as transparent in on-the-ground contexts as they were in the United States and Caribbean,[4] though similar patriarchal barriers emerged. Titi (Nigeria chapter leader), a goat and ram herder, and Lydia (Ghana chapter leader), an

[4] Race has played a significant role in the colonial histories that have constructed the current social conditions in Africa, but is not as transparent in daily on-the-ground contexts due to the racial homogeneity of many African countries.

organic fruit and vegetable farmer, discussed how women in Africa were often overlooked and underacknowledged for their contributions to farming and supporting community food security by male leaders in agriculture, despite being responsible for the majority of farm production labor.

> ...despite their contribution to global food security, women farming [sic] are frequently underestimated and overlooked in this area. Men dominance [sic] in decision making, in housing, and all those economic as well as agricultural production has continued to oppress we women. Even though we are the key producer of labor, we have not been recognized enough.
>
> As it is, we have at least 70% women according to statistics, at least 70% women involved in agriculture. The greater labor force is from the women, yes. It's only unfortunate [sic] that we do not get to access what we need in order to be productive.
>
> (*LYDIA*)

These barriers represented a mere cross-section of relational challenges the women experienced in their quest to access resources and community in agriculture, pushing many of them to the brink of giving up farming altogether. Feeling lost and disconnected from their agrarian and cultural heritage, meeting other ACB women through NWIAA's network was a serendipitous lifeline for many of the participants to foster connection to a diasporic sisterhood and renew their purpose for farming as a form of resistance and supporting local and global community food security efforts.

## Conclusion

By zooming in and out to offer intersecting snapshots of Tammy's family history with some of the interpersonal experiences of NWIAA chapter leaders, this chapter brought together additional on-the-ground context to situate the contemporary social conditions ACB women farmers face. The ethnographic research detailed the wide-ranging challenges ACB communities must navigate to combat their political disenfranchisement, while simultaneously shining a light on the transformative potential of large-scale solutions such as land reform as viable and sustainable public health responses. At the same time, the deep analysis of participants' micro-level, everyday stories of intersectional discrimination drew attention to how embedded patriarchy and racism in agriculture upheld existing power inequities even as the women gained access to resources and leadership positions.

The Steele family "40 acres" narrative emerges within a political landscape marked by peak levels of polarization, where the extreme divide has forced ideas previously deemed centrist to shift to one side of the proverbial spectrum. While the conservative right has successfully mainstreamed prior insupportable conversations around topics of reproductive rights, gun ownership, and immigration, simultaneously the progressive left has platformed ideas once thought of as radical (e.g., reparations, land reform) in a way not seen since the period directly post-Civil War. As referenced above, the 2020 social crises birthed several revolutionary bill proposals and task forces to study the potentiality of reparations by politicians and lawmakers. Despite the subsequent "whitelash" and lost momentum that emerged in response to many of these deliberations, public health leaders have largely remained consistent in their efforts to keep reparations conversations in the forefront, undeterred by the subsiding political momentum. However, conspicuously missing from these efforts were leaders in the agricultural sector.

For example, in the time since 2020, policy conversations around equity in agriculture have been careful not to explicitly mention the word "reparations" in government discourse for fear of political backlash (Wallance, 2021). Instead, they have primarily implemented provisional initiatives such as the USDA Discrimination Financial Assistance Program that incorporate more immediate, short-term solutions such as one-time payouts. Indeed, such approaches are meaningful and symbolic gestures to account for past transgressions, however, they are limited in scope as they address only one component of ACB land and farm loss (Daniel, 1985; Litwack, 2009). While early Reconstruction policies were more holistic in their approach toward social equity (e.g., aligning across multiple sectors and social determinant categories), decisions to focus on reductionist and segmented solutions (e.g., cash payments) to the crisis halted important progress toward transformative change and limited the scope of problem definition and solution(s). Further, by not directly engaging discussions on reparations, agricultural policymakers miss an important opportunity to build upon multilevel, upstream solutions with other sectors, such as public health.

Such reductionist logics also emerge when discussing the importance of access. As described above, many public health practitioners and interventionists posit *access* as a key factor in determining health and social outcomes. To support their assertion, they draw on a large body of research that points to *lack of* access as the primary catalyst for upholding inequities across diverse health contexts (Andrulis, 1998; Riley, 2012; Srivastav et al., 2020). While an essential first step, emerging counter evidence complicates these beliefs to demonstrate *that access alone is not enough* to foster fair and equitable social conditions. For example, an extensive body of health communication research exploring interactions in patient-provider settings has demonstrated that members from marginalized groups are often met with additional challenges even *after* gaining access to the healthcare system, citing discordances in language barriers, culturally concordant care, and health literacy (Kim et al., 2021; Terui et al., 2023). More related to the context of this book, interdisciplinary food security research found that simply providing access to healthy food options (e.g., farmers markets, community supported agriculture programs, healthy corner store initiatives, incentive programs) is often not enough to foster equitable conditions among marginalized populations, as they often overlook broader cultural and structural influences such as culturally relevant foods, whiteness in alternative and charity food spaces, and lack of leadership among people-of-color in such spaces (see Babb et al., 2023; Conrad & Zuckerman, 2020; de Souza, 2019; Larimore, 2018).

Paralleling these examples, the participants' self-described interpersonal barriers demonstrate how it is not enough to simply create access for ACB women to become equitable in agriculture. As evidenced across many of the women's stories, several already held influential leadership positions, were highly educated (45 percent of participants completed graduate school; 36 percent graduated from college; 9 percent attended some college), and regularly engaged with leaders in dominant agricultural spaces. In his popular TED Talk, Boston University professor Dr. Anthony Jack stated "access ain't inclusion" when describing the inequitable conditions for Black students navigating Predominantly White Institutions in the United States. In agriculture, providing ACB women access to a toxic system that strips them of their cultural assets, does not take them seriously, and simultaneously co-opts and extracts their knowledge will not generate the radical reenvisioning of possibilities required to enact transformative change, and in many ways obscures the root causes of the problem. To demonstrate how the women of NWIAA navigated these multilevel challenges, the next chapter introduces "politics of resourcefulness" as a guiding heuristic for understanding their generative strategies against dominant "resilience" discourses.

# 4

## From Grassroots to Grasstops

### Taking Up Space, Seeking Sisterhood, and External Allies

TO UNDERSTAND HOW AFRICAN, CARIBBEAN, and Black (ACB) women farmers navigate inequitable social structures while protecting and advancing their cultural legacies, historical lived experiences, and shared deep-rooted agricultural knowledge, this chapter applies two axioms of POR, *resources* and *recognition*, to the corpus of ethnographic data. As discussed in the introduction of this book, dominant public health intervention approaches to addressing food insecurity are often located within existing knowledge hierarchies that simultaneously work to privilege certain cause-effect rationales and tools used to measure and define problems while simultaneously limiting the agency of "targeted" local communities by framing them from a deficit lens in need of resources and knowledge from power brokers outside of the community. These models are often undergirded by a capitalist logic that works to segment geographic resources and cultural assets and erase local meanings around food, farming, and land (Breilh, 2021; Dutta, 2020). Embedded under the guise of humanitarianism, local communities are left to remain "resilient" and adaptable to existing social and political conditions—paradoxically, by the very interventions seeking to mitigate the issues.

*Seeds of Sovereignty*. Andrew L. Carter, Oxford University Press. © Oxford University Press (2026).
DOI: 10.1093/9780197789391.003.0004

An antidote to disrupting "deficit" models and resilience discourses in dominant public health approaches requires adopting the counter-hegemonic vision where local communities can engage in democratic dialogue and create alternative agendas that contest mainstream logics (Derickson, 2016). Given *POR*'s specific focus on interrogating existing social relations, resourceful models draw attention to the need for communities to be recognized *externally* by political actors who can support structural change (e.g., redistribution efforts) and "recognition towards a vision of resourceful communities" (Mackinnon & Derickson, 2013, p. 263). Additionally, communities must also be recognized *internally* by in-group stakeholders who engender "a sense of confidence, self-worth, and community affirmation" that can be used to "fuel the mobilization of existing resources and argue for and pursue new resources" (Mackinnon & Derickson, 2013, p. 265).

This chapter comprises two primary sections. The first section introduces *resources* as an experiential guide for public health practitioners and communities to identify and privilege local and cultural assets. Through this application, it documents how the women of NWIAA used resources as a *POR* strategy to create material and discursive conditions to come together, "take up" physical and intellectual space, cultivate voice infrastructures, and forge weak-tie partnerships outside of mainstream agricultural spaces and traditions. The second section of the chapter establishes *recognition* as a guiding public health praxis for documenting structural inequities and state culpability. By applying this axiom, it documents the resourcefulness strategies participants used to engender external and internal recognition from both top-down power brokers and in-group community stakeholders, and how these actions were constrained by the complex, sociopolitical conditions that undergirded them—particularly in relation to their precarious social positions as ACB women.

## Resources

On the morning of September 21, 2023, two chartered buses pulled up in succession to an adjacent parking lot across from the US Capitol Building. Minutes later, the Capitol lawn was soddened by a sea of people wearing pink shirts that read in stylized text: "*From Fields to Futures: Empowering Women Uplifting Children and Breaking Poverty.*" After receiving the proverbial marching orders from protest organizers, the mass of folks quickly assembled into marching lines and made their way along the famed Constitution Avenue. Led in formation by grassroots activist Porsche "Queen" Miller and a cavalcade of NWIAA chapter leaders and members, and various celebrities and politicians, including WNBA Hall-of-Famer Ruthie Bolton (Mississippi chapter leader), American music executive Eddie Levert Jr., Lieutenant Governor of Vermont David Zuckerman, among other local community activists, the "Equity and Inclusion" protest march brought important attention to the plight of ACB women farmers and generated support for NWIAA to become the first ever Black congressionally chartered organization in the United States. Making stops at the Capitol Building, USDA Headquarters, and the White House and flanked by a coordinated police escort, the event was an impactful sign of unity among the ACB women farming community and sent a murmur across the D.C. political landscape (See Figures 4.1, 4.2, and 4.3).

Most observably, the "Equity and Inclusion" march exemplified NWIAA's ability to foster community networks, build infrastructure, and bring together seemingly disparate groups of people. After grabbing my protest sign that read "Black Women Have Solutions to Poverty Issues!" I quickly assumed my position in line, eager to begin the march and lend my voice in solidarity. In between unified chants such as "Show me what community looks like...This is what community looks like!" and "When our children are under attack, what do we do? Stand up fight back!" I engaged in several conversations with marchers as they described what drew them to be involved with NWIAA and their motivations for attending the protest. During our stop for lunch at the Department of Agriculture Headquarters food hall, I sat next to Noreen (US Georgia chapter leader), one of the organization's original six-chapter leaders, who excitedly shared her farming origin story and inspiration for mobilizing Black women farmers and youth. Noreen was a dignitary in the Black farming community writ large, known for her ability to bring together people in the US South and across the country. As evidence of her organizing prowess, she single-handedly assembled thirty members from her NWIAA Georgia chapter (Georgia Women

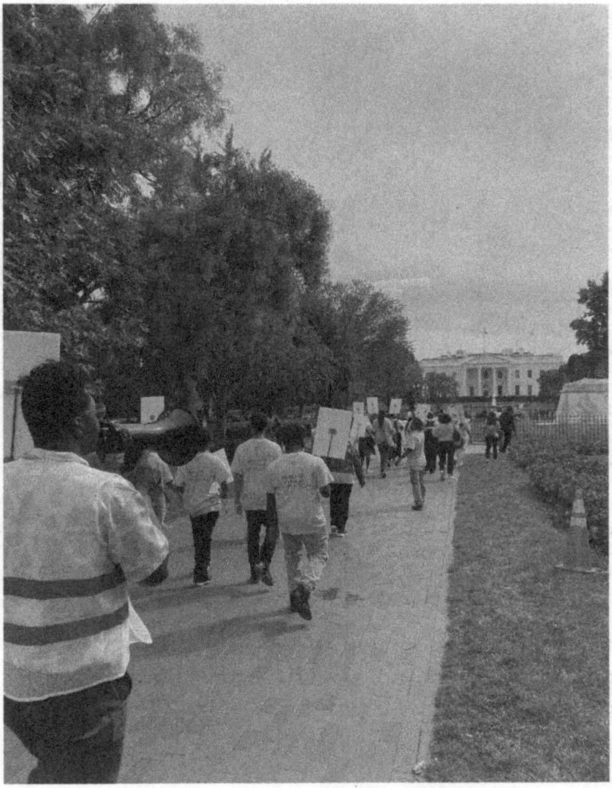

FIGURE 4.1 NWIAA marchers walking to the White House lawn.
Photo by author

in Agriculture Association; GWIAA) to attend the protest. When I asked Noreen about how she was able to bring so many people together, she simply replied, "I'm a connector of people. So I kind of connected some things together."

Noreen's ethos as a "connector" is reflective of how NWIAA offers a space for women to come together. As referenced in the previous chapters, ACB women farmers' political voice, lived experience, and unique agricultural skill sets have largely been erased and disconnected from one another in mainstream agriculture discourses and other health-promoting initiatives, such as the alternative food and critical agrarian movements—which has led many ACB women to feel isolated and internalize their own purported demise (Ramirez, 2015).

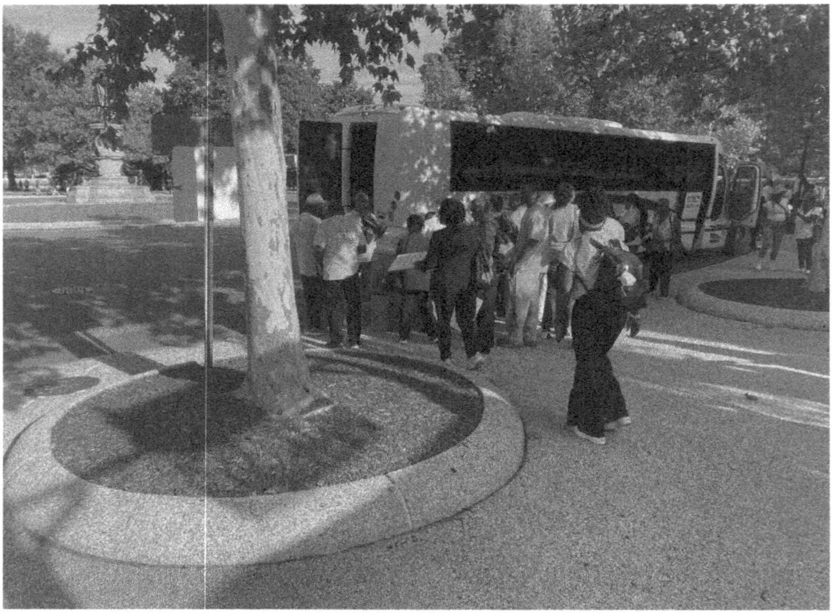

FIGURE 4.2 Marchers receiving instruction on their scheduled route shortly after arriving in front of the US Capitol building.
Photo by author

Thus, creating the material and social conditions for ACB women farmers to come together, render themselves visible, and "take up" space is an important first step to restoring ACB community foodways (Carter et al., 2024; Layman & Civita, 2022).

## Bringing Women Together and Becoming Visible

Like some of the reactions I received from my professional colleagues when learning about the scope and impact of ACB women farmers, many of the participants were similarly shocked at the extent of remaining women actively working in agriculture before their involvement with NWIAA. Vivian (Tennessee chapter leader) was introduced to farming at a young age through herding livestock and growing crops on her aunt and uncle's farm in West Alabama. Upon graduating from high school, she moved to Knoxville, Tennessee, vowing to leave farming behind forever after becoming disheartened by its arduous nature and the

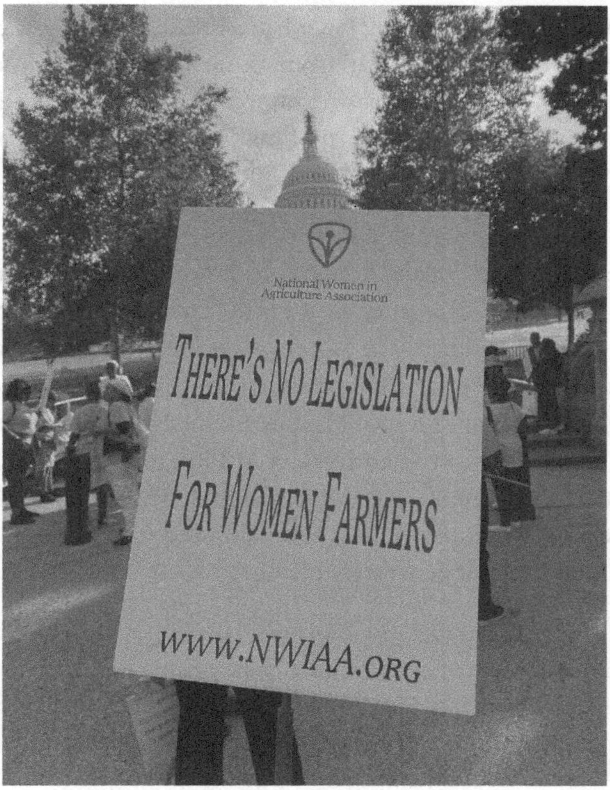
National Women in
Agriculture Association
THERE'S NO LEGISLATION
FOR WOMEN FARMERS
WWW.NWIAA.ORG

FIGURE 4.3 A protest sign at the "Equity and Inclusion" march.
Photo by author

scant long-term opportunities offered to women like her. However, she had a change of heart in 2010, when she attended a national NWIAA conference after her cousin convinced her to attend (who had been working with the organization at the time). Shortly after attending the conference and meeting some of the women involved, her passion to pursue agriculture was restored once again. During our conversation, she reflected on inspirational feelings after seeing so many ambitious ACB women with similar levels of knowledge and expertise as herself.

> You meet some very, very successful women in agriculture and farming in this organization, because my first experience of meeting someone, I met a lady when we were in Tuskegee. She had a chicken

> farm. And then another lady I met had a blueberry farm. And it was just exciting to see women with something like that. And I thought, 'Oh, my gosh, I didn't know women were even doing stuff like this myself.' But it's a thing where you find a lot of smart and ambitious women in National Women in Agriculture.

Several other participants described feeling inspired and a renewed sense of purpose to farm and support community food security efforts after seeing other ACB women farmers in leadership roles. For Bridget (Arizona chapter leader), the combined challenges of accessing resources, low political power, and limited exposure to other Black people in agriculture was enough to make her seriously question her capacity to continue farming in the arid desert of Phoenix, Arizona. However, after joining NWIAA in 2021 and participating in their weekly chapter leader check-in meetings, she felt reinvigorated to mobilize with other ACB women to foster generative change.

> I mean, being a part of just their weekly web meeting and seeing so many women farmers was just amazing. It just blew my mind. And Black women, too. So it encouraged me to continue. Because it's tough. You could be out here, and it's just you literally on this half acre, and you're growing food, and to know that it's a whole movement going on out there that is in flow with it. And that's the NWIAA.

Many of the participants discussed how not having a social network prevented them from seeking help and advice when they were in a bind or needed to find out information, but being a part of a broader community helped them feel seen and heard. Crystal (Rhode Island chapter leader) became interested in the business side of farming as a second career when the realities of COVID-19 forced her to critically think about the importance of growing food and land ownership, where she first collaborated with NWIAA to provide grant writing support. Before her partnership, she felt invisible after getting repeatedly shut out from the USDA and other dominant power brokers when asking for information or clarifying questions, driving her to almost give up on farming before she could learn the ins and outs of the industry. However, after being connected to NWIAA through a mutual third party, she quickly established a sense of trust and support, which kept her motivated to continue. When I asked her to characterize the organization as possessing a core set of values, she talked about their willingness to help and provide visibility to anyone in need, which was an important personal virtue.

> I know it's the National *Women* in Agriculture, but anyone that comes to the table, anyone that wants help, man, woman, child, they're there. So they're just caring. They just bring a lot to the table. They're just there. Anyone that needs anything, they're going to be helpful. And I've reached out to other organizations here. We have a local place—even calling my local USDA office, no one called me back. But I can call the NWIAA, and they're going to call, pick up the phone, and they're going to call someone at one of the offices or whatever, or whoever they know. And they'll get back, and they get me on the phone.
>
> (*CRYSTAL*)

For Crystal, simple care ethics such as finding someone who was reliable to reach on the phone was enough to keep her grounded in her purpose to farm. Selena (North Carolina chapter leader) similarly discussed how she felt excluded and ignored by external gatekeepers when asking for information or general guidance, which led her to the organization.

> When I keep getting doors shut in my face, or rejection letters, or not right now, or emails that's not opened or returned, and things like that, it's kind of like who is trying to help me reach my goal? I mean, even down to—I'll make a phone call, and it's returned by an intern that I don't even know. I'm like, 'Who is trying to help me reach my goals?' ... that's one of the things that brought me to NWIAA—and I've tried not to be that—I don't want to be seen as a troublemaker.

Selena's narrative builds on the deep sense of alienation and overlooked needs that many ACB women farmers experience. Moreover, her concern with being labeled as a "troublemaker" further reinforces double consciousness feelings, drawing attention to the delicate balance ACB women must strike between voicing their legitimate grievances and navigating the threat of racist and patriarchal discrimination that can undermine their credibility and efforts at any point.

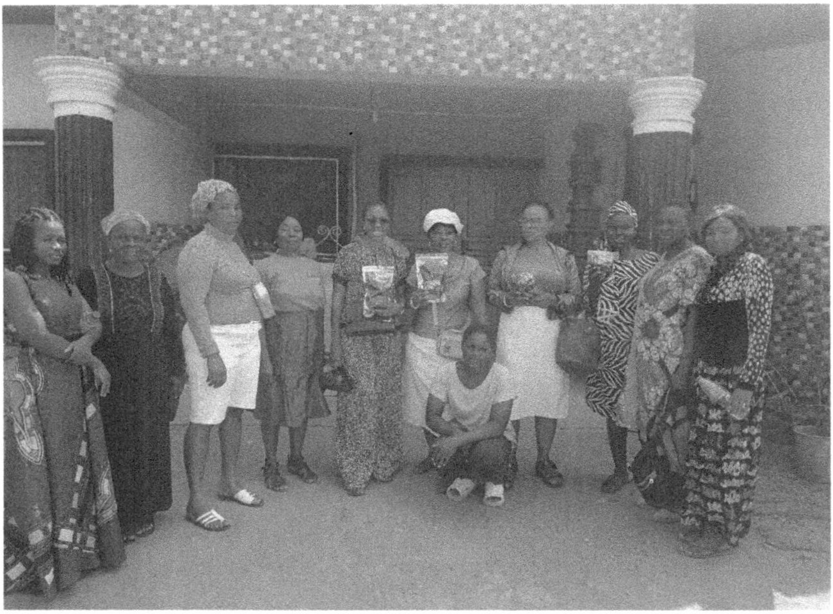

**FIGURE 4.4** Betty (Nigeria chapter leader; center left) at the NWIAA Africa country representative training in Lagos, Nigeria.
Photo by Olaitan Ariyo

Mainstream narratives frame ACB farmers (and ACB women, specifically) as a dwindling and nearly extinct population due to their lack of education about how to farm, own (and pass down) land, and mobilize political power; though, it is often an accumulation of the daily, microlevel frustrations such as those described by Crystal and Selena, that if properly addressed early enough, could mitigate (and restore) diminished investment among these groups. Other women, such as Juhna (Missouri chapter leader) and Betty (Nigeria chapter leader), a fish and aquaculture farmer and president of the collective NWIAA Africa chapters, described how NWIAA provided a space to explore leadership roles, platform their voice, and shine a light on the work of other transnational ACB women (see Figure 4.4).

> [NWIAA] just had all these things that they were doing, all these wonderful things. I've seen [other state chapter leaders] that look like me in positions, and I said, you know what? I want to be there... And they offered me the chance to be that chairperson in Missouri, to be

> that resource. Because like I said, when you go anywhere, you need an umbrella. Because the underdog sometimes get tired of fighting by themselves, that's why some wolves run in a pack because I cannot take over the whole world by myself.
>
> (JUHNA)

> If you want your voice to be heard, if you want what you do to be felt, not only by the people among the people, but globally, then you have to join [NWIAA] because that is what it is to me. It opens your eyes to so many opportunities, opportunities that you were blind to. Your eyes are being open to it right even in your country. You don't even have to go to the US.
>
> (BETTY)

Juhna's analogy of wolves running in a pack identifies how lonely (and dangerous) it can be for ACB women to be siloed and disconnected from other interlocutors and underscores the importance of community connection to provide protection and support to resist conditions of gendered capitalism that position them in segmented factions to compete for resources. Relatedly, Betty's excerpt draws attention to the power of transnational collaboration for making "hidden" opportunities and partnerships visible.

### Cultivating Alternative Communication Infrastructures

> *NWIAA is here with your Women In Ag Wednesday Talk Show December 2022 Schedule! Don't forget to grab your favorite healthy snack and listen to the Agmazing stories we have to share.*

This caption was posted to NWIAA's Instagram page on December 1, 2022. The post highlighted the docket of guests scheduled to appear on its "Women in Ag Wednesdays" YouTube talk show (see Figure 4.5). NWIAA incorporates a host of online social media platforms to center the voices of Black women leaders and youth in agriculture.[1] In a social and political climate where ACB women farmers are not descriptively

[1] The NWIAA headquarters social media accounts include 26.8K followers on Instagram, 1.5K followers on X, 42.3K followers on Facebook, and 264 followers on YouTube.

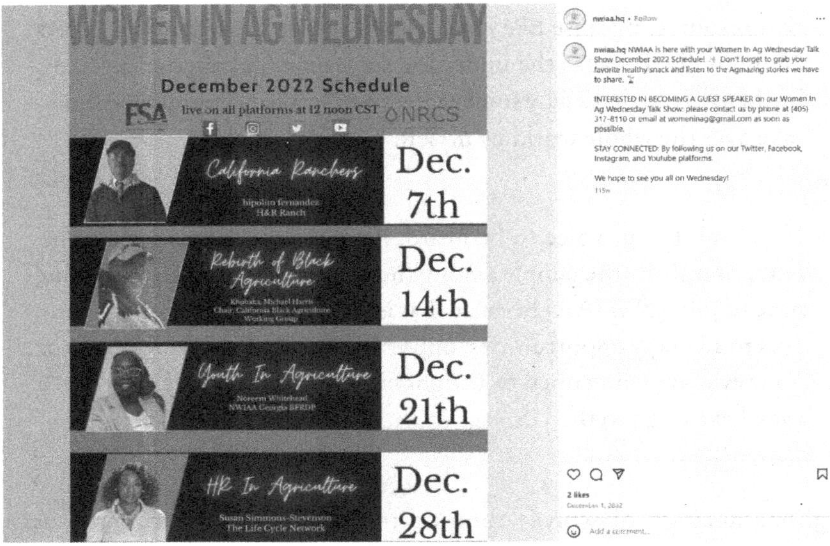
WOMEN IN AG WEDNESDAY
December 2022 Schedule
FSA
live on all platforms at 12 noon CST
NRCS
California Ranchers
Dec. 7th
Rebirth of Black Agriculture
Dec. 14th
Youth In Agriculture
Dec. 21th
HR In Agriculture
Dec. 28th
nwiaa.hq • Follow
nwiaa.hq NWIAA is here with your Women In Ag Wednesday Talk Show December 2022 Schedule! Don't forget to grab your favorite healthy snack and listen to the Agmazing stories we have to share.
INTERESTED IN BECOMING A GUEST SPEAKER on our Women In Ag Wednesday Talk Show: please contact us by phone at (405) 317-8110 or email at womeninag@gmail.com as soon as possible.
STAY CONNECTED: By following us on our Twitter, Facebook, Instagram, and Youtube platforms.
We hope to see you all on Wednesday!
2 likes

**FIGURE 4.5** Instagram post promoting Women in Ag Wednesday, December 2022 guest schedule.

nor substantively represented in the cultural memory of mainstream society, the creation and dissemination of the weekly talk show allowed them to carve out embedded communication spaces to recapture community agency and share information with one another in a way that is transparent and trustworthy (Hayes & Hibbing, 2017).

A vital component of making subaltern communities visible to the public involves creating access to alternative infrastructures that exist outside of mainstream media platforms that incentivize their participation in decision-making and knowledge creation processes (Dutta et al., 2016). Critical health communication scholar Mohan Dutta highlights the importance of such groups developing alternative communication platforms, such as community-driven media channels, advocacy campaigns, and local performances, as a mechanism for creating spaces where historically disenfranchised voices can disrupt marginalizing structures and reshape cultural narratives (Dutta, 2018). In the context of *POR*, the development of alternative communication infrastructures allows local communities to "have the [material and discursive] capacity to engage in genuinely deliberative democratic dialogue to develop contestable alternative agendas and work in ways that meaningfully challenge existing power relations," an important step for challenging reductionist "resilience" discourses popular in public health and agriculture that extract group agency via deficit-driven intervention models (MacKinnon & Derickson, 2013, p. 263). As such, NWIAA and its stakeholders built community capacity by co-creating alternative communication platforms that were meaningful and relevant to them.

The women identified multiple ways that developing voice infrastructures was integral for them to network transnationally with other ACB women farmers, receive exposure for their businesses, obtain relevant information and resources, and politically mobilize as a collective. Communication platforms such as the monthly chapter leader meetings (a virtual event for all chapter leaders and members [US, USVI, Africa]) to provide two-way updates and receive general support), themed conferences, annual training workshops, youth summits, and various social media channels were incorporated to foster spaces of engagement that participants perceived as safe for receiving and disseminating information and subverting top-down intervention messaging. In some African contexts, unique histories of gendered capitalism have prevented women from accessing trustworthy information and passing it down to other local farmers (Mudege et al., 2017; Tsige et al., 2020). Betty (Nigeria chapter leader) and Lydia (Ghana chapter leader) discussed how such alternative infrastructures helped them navigate these challenges (see Figure 4.6).

> That is one of the benefits of collaboration, it brings women together to collaborate... You talk to women. You're getting to see information, good information on how you can do your thing if it did not work this way, good information. That information, when it comes to me, I pass it down to the grassroot farmer because that's really my aim. I just want the minority farmers to be included in whatever the government is doing, in whatever we are doing, so that it can make money for the farmer and it can be impactful in their community.
>
> *(BETTY)*

> Most of the times, we do have our monthly meetings via Google Teams. So through that, our [chapter leaders] from all states, we gather and share ideas. We gather to learn from each other. 'What

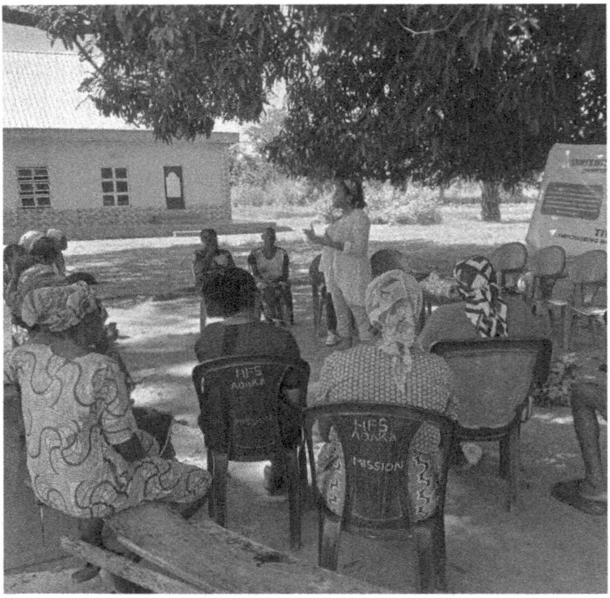

**FIGURE 4.6** NWIAA Africa chapter leader training on sweet potato cultivation in Benue State, Nigeria.

Photo by Olaitan Ariyo

> other practices are you doing, that we can learn from each other?' And we have capacity building...We train ourselves on knowledge sharing and how to improve—how to add technology into our farming. So that is basically what we normally do. So [our group] has really benefited from [NWIAA] through trainings and other stuff.
>
> (*LYDIA*)

Since many of the women felt ignored and overlooked when reaching out individually to food and agriculture administrators and related offices and acquire new information, NWIAA created platforms to bring resources and support from top-down entities directly to the women by circumventing red-tape barriers (e.g., gathering enough women to meet baseline quotas for organizations such as USDA and NRCS to provide information booths at NWIAA conferences) and drawing on its own diverse networks and partnerships. For example, in 2023, when the National Black Farmers Association (one of the leading Black farming advocacy groups in the United States) was looking to promote their workshops across the country to bring awareness to the $2.2 billion Inflation Reduction Act discrimination suit, they reached out to various NWIAA chapter sites to host the events, knowing their capacity to develop alternative communication infrastructures and as a trusted interlocutor in the Black farming community. In 2024, NWIAA hosted various virtual "Resource and Equity" summits where a live USDA and NRCS representative answered questions and provided information regarding their sponsored programs to chapter leaders and members. In Nigeria, several NWIAA Africa chapters facilitated partnerships with the Rivers State Ministry of Agriculture and USAID to hold several "train-the-trainer" events, where they participated in training sessions to teach different farming and growing techniques to NWIAA chapter leaders for them to disseminate to their local members.

Highlighting the multiple strategies NWIAA used to bring collective resources to their stakeholders not available to them individually is important to underscore from an intervention perspective, though, as noted in the previous chapter, access alone is not a panacea and draws attention to the complexities low-resourced communities face in their capacity to acquire relevant resources. For instance, some of the programs referenced by the participants, such as the "train-the-trainer" events and USDA information sessions, often employ outside "experts" to create the curriculum and disseminate the training/workshops. This process positions the women as empty vessels open for receiving new information. Often left out of these programs are conversations about the women's unique assets and skillsets (e.g., local growing practices, cultural knowledge) and how they can be integrated within existing knowledge frameworks. Further, as these trainings are often carried out in-kind at no or reduced cost, there is often a built-in assumption that the participants will adopt certain practices or growing techniques when disseminating the information to their members—in the process obscuring many of their own embedded cultural assets. Widespread interdisciplinary critical work has interrogated the structural mechanisms and outreach strategies of top-down NGOs and government entities such as the United States Agency for International Development (USAID), USDA, Food and Agriculture Organization of the United Nations, and the Bill and Melinda Gates Foundation for simultaneously garnering community support and maintaining control of food governance processes, particularly in Africa and Global South contexts (Borras & Mohamed, 2020; Canfield, 2022).

## Forging "Weak-Tie" Partnerships

Given how ACB women farmers are largely erased from mainstream communication platforms, many of the participants were burdened with the dual undertaking of making themselves relevant and visible to top-down power brokers (e.g., making sure their numbers were counted in the USDA Census of Agriculture reports, having enough representative research and scientific evidence of their impact to justify receiving grant monies and political support), while simultaneously searching in the "proverbial dark" for similar ACB women to quell their own internalized feelings of isolation and reinforce their resolve to continue farming. Regarding the latter—it is remarkable the extent to which ACB women have impacted farming and agriculture globally with such a fractured and decentralized network. For many of the participants, arguably the biggest resource NWIAA fostered was not in its direct connections cultivated among other members and chapter leaders across the broader organizational network, but in its ability to foster "weak tie" partnerships with other ACB women from disparate communities and networks outside of their own. In this way, the mere bringing of women together galvanized the participants to seek out other partnerships and opportunities—even with a scarcity of power and resources—to allay their "far, few, in-between" perceptions and prompt the more fundamental question: *how impactful could these capacity-building and organizing efforts be with actual large-scale political support and sustainable resources*?

Stanford sociologist Mark Granovetter proposed his "strength of weak ties" theory (1973) to suggest that weak social ties, or casual connections and loose acquaintances, play an integral role in disseminating information and opportunities within social networks. Granovetter argues that weak ties act as bridges between different social groups, allowing information and opportunities to flow across broader networks. He posits that close ties, such as family and friend networks, tend to form dense clusters of similar people, leading to the distribution of repetitive information; while weak ties connect disparate and seemingly unrelated clusters to bring in new information and opportunities. Other key components to Granovetter's theory include access to novel information and unique opportunities, social mobility, and maximizing social capital.

In the context of ACB women farmers, an exploration of weak-tie connections is a useful way for understanding how marginalized communities generate social capital and essential support, particularly against the backdrop of historical subjugation and limited access to privileged "hidden" communication networks that uphold the status quo. Many of the participants mentioned the various collaborations and partnerships they made through informal, casual interconnections outside of dominant social networks and their strong tie communities. Selena (US South Carolina chapter) described an example where she was discovered by another women's farming organization to serve as a keynote speaker at their conference through a weak tie connection.

> Just recently, last week, I've been invited to be a keynote speaker at Blue Ridge Women in Ag Association Conference. And they found me through National Women in Ag Facebook—I mean, through their page. And so that right there is huge. So when [NWIAA] put us out there representing the organization, then, I mean, that goes back to making those outreach connections because Blue Ridge—they're in the mountains, Boone, North Carolina. So being able to be seen and heard by your peers that look like you is going to be huge.

Selena's weak ties fostered via an ancillary social media connection allowed her to access new opportunities (keynote speaker) which most likely would not have materialized through her strong ties, who often share overlapping and duplicative opportunities. Moreover, her articulation of "being able to be seen and heard by your peers that look like you" symbolizes how weak ties can amplify hidden voices and create outreach connections that may not have been possible with a more closed, strong-tie network.

Weak tie associations also allowed participants to bring together disparate people and institutions. For example, Noreen (US Georgia chapter leader) and a former Mississippi chapter leader received a grant from the USDA National Institute of Food and Agriculture's Beginning Farmer and Rancher Development Program to teach women with no agricultural experience how to farm. The program brought together stakeholders from Fort Valley State University (an HBCU located in central Georgia), the University of Georgia, and local community members. By combining their unique assets and skill sets (Noreen as a connector of people, the Mississippi chapter leader as an agricultural expert), they "bridged" social capital by allowing members from different social groups to share ideas and experiences with new and diverse audiences (Putnam, 2000). Noreen detailed the process of how they spearheaded the collaboration during our conversation (see Figure 4.7).

> I placed all of our chapter—not all of them, but a good number of the chapter members in a program. A beginner farmer program that was dealing with herbs and medicinal hemp. And so the next year, [the Mississippi chapter leader] saw that I can get people in a program. So she said, 'Well, let's do a beginner farm program together.' I said, 'Yeah.' And so we did. And she did it in Mississippi, and I did

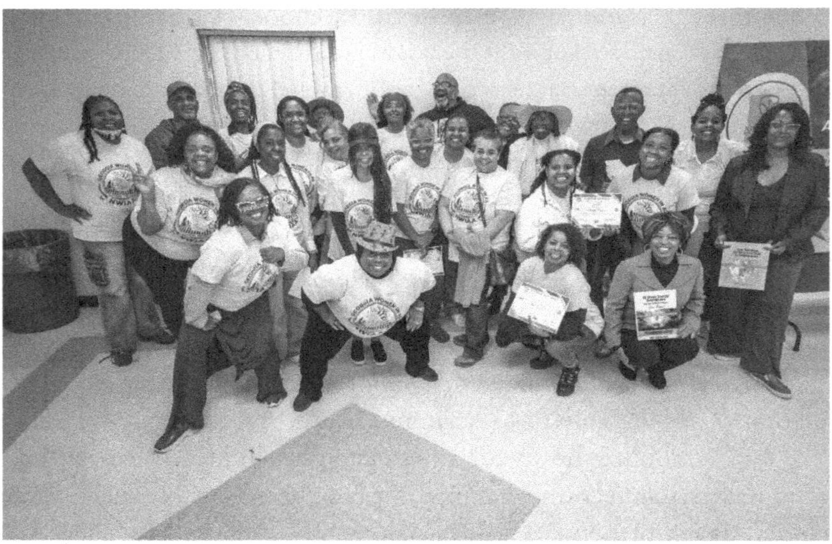

**FIGURE 4.7** NWIAA Georgia (GWIAA) Beginning Farmer and Rancher Development Program graduating cohort.

Photo by Noreen Whitehead

> it [in Georgia]. So we're kind of like bouncing off of each other. I'm bouncing off of her because she's more experienced than I am. I just know how to get all the people to what you're doing. And she does the other part piece to it. So we kind of work hand-in-hand. So she just needed access to the people. She already had the information. So when you know how to work—when you have a good partner that you mesh together in what you're doing, there's not going to be any issues. And so we were able to make a program happen. And she knew all the UGA, University of Georgia, people. And I knew the people over at Fort Valley. So we always work hand-in-hand like that.

Like Noreen and the former Mississippi chapter leader, several other participants discussed how being involved with NWIAA created new opportunities for them to merge weak ties with their own initiatives or inspired them to create their own. For Betty (Nigeria chapter leader) and Diana (USVI chapter leader), weak tie associations allowed them to connect seemingly disparate groups of people together and fostered a sense of urgency for them to intensify their advocacy efforts.

> I feel that [NWIAA] are going to help my movement, like partnering with Ministry of Agriculture, partnering with what we call Girl Power Initiative. It's an organization where they have girls, and they train them. So it's like a wake-up call. That's the word. It's like a wake-up call for me, for me to be on my toes and get things done because seriously, we have a long way to go, a long way.
>
> *(BETTY)*

> There were female farmers I used to talk to for years on the phone, via email, and like one in Alabama, one in DC, and one in Toronto. And we've been talking for years. And it's only this year that we committed to meeting, and two of them came [to St. Croix]. The one from D.C. and Alabama came here and did some work for me on my—because I had a torn rotator cuff and I did surgery, and I was kind of limb for a while. And I just got this house and I needed a hand. And they came for a week and we now are doing things. And out of that, I started to think about doing the Woman in Agriculture, Virgin Islands Women in Agriculture chapter, because one of them knows about [NWIAA's] National Chapter. That's how things are built when you interact and you network and communicate, and

> that's what we need to encourage more in farming. Black farmers don't know other Black farmers. That's the problem. And the white farmers aren't helping no Black farmers.
>
> (*DIANA*)

As a social resource, weak tie partnerships served different goals and fulfilled different needs for the women depending on their geosocial contexts. For the United States and US Caribbean chapter leaders and members, weak ties allowed them to access new opportunities and connect with previously unknown allies and like-minded groups to help combat their extinction status in the US food system. For NWIAA Africa stakeholders, weak tie associations connected them to access new resources and seek US-based grant monies and programs previously unavailable to them without a US partner.

## Recognition

In the 2020 US Presidential election, President Biden was victorious over incumbent Donald Trump, marking one of the most politically and culturally polarizing decisions in decades. As political analysts dissected the results in the months following the election, a key reason why Biden was victorious was due to the overwhelming support of Black voters, particularly Black women, with 95 percent of them casting their vote in his favor. In his acceptance speech, Biden told Black voters that he would repay their loyalty by having *their* backs like they had his (Hall, 2020). In the years following Biden's political victory, Black women waited enduringly for him to come through on his promise, to varying degrees of approval. This exercise of holding Biden's proverbial feet to the fire is reflective of Black women's rich history seeking recognition from government leaders for their political power and sociocultural influence (Farmer, 2017; Jones, 2020). During NWIAA's "Equity and Inclusion" protest, marchers drew directly from these intertextual discourses as they prepared signs that read "President Biden, Help Us as We Helped You!" and synchronized chants of "President Biden, save our children!"

As referenced above, an integral step toward a *POR* praxis requires communities to be recognized both *externally* and *internally.*

This section documents the resourcefulness strategies NWIAA employed to engender external and internal recognition, highlighting the complex sociopolitical conditions that informed their actions.

### External Recognition

Less than one month after the "Equity and Inclusion" protest, NWIAA leadership was invited back to Washington D.C., this time to provide testimony to members from the White House policy council in support of their proposal to become a congressionally chartered organization and serve as a pilot program of 4-H (a US-based network of organizations that develop citizenship, leadership, responsibility, and life skills of youth through experiential learning and a positive youth development approach) for Black women and youth in agriculture. In the organization's fifteen-plus years of mobilizing efforts, this was the closest they had come to realizing their goal of securing sustainable government funding for ACB women farmers.

During the scheduled date of the White House briefing, I happened to be in town for an academic conference across the Potomac River in neighboring National Harbor, Maryland, where I was asked by NWIAA leadership to attend the briefing and provide testimony based on my research and multi-year academic-community partnership with the organization. After congregating outside of the White House's Eisenhower Building, we made our way through the high-security metal detector, where we received our temporary visitor badges and were escorted to the conference room where the presentation would take place. Over the next 30 minutes, members from the leadership team presented prepared remarks in support of their proposed bill. Additionally, several industry and political stakeholders called in to the meeting via phone to give testimony on the organization's behalf, including former US representatives and members from various agriculture lobbying groups.

Since its inception in 2008, NWIAA has adopted a multilevel approach in its advocacy efforts by combining both grassroots (bottom-up, collective community-level mobilizing) and grasstops (top-down, outreach via targeted decision makers) organizing models (Grefe, 1997; see Figure 4.8). As a case study for exploring the nuances of *how* and

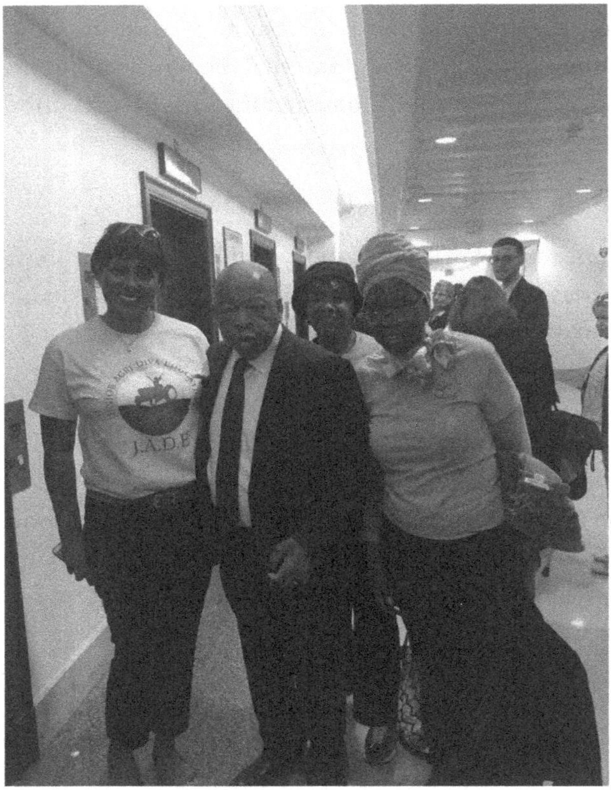


**FIGURE 4.8** *From right to left*: Georgia chapter leader Noreen, Tennessee chapter leader Vivian, civil rights icon and former Georgia Congressperson John Lewis, and Tammy at the NWIAA 10th year Celebration of Minority Female Farmers Saving At-Risk-Youth on Capitol Hill in Washington, D.C., during Black History Month, February 27, 2018.

Photo by Noreen Whitehead

*why* low-power communities navigate structural barriers to engage in public health and food justice activism, the women of NWIAA offer many unique insights. As noted throughout the empirical chapters in this book, many of the participants were keenly aware of their low-power status and precarious social position vis-a-vis local and national policymakers, which bound them to a double consciousness reality of having to go through traditional channels of power that did not threaten dominant structures and worked within existing rules and laws. On the other hand, their mere positionalities as ACB women and core motivations for food justice organizing (i.e., centering ACB women's lived experience and shared knowledge in food system ideology, supporting local and global ACB community food security projects) were fundamentally radical and upset hegemonic assumptions about who gets to participate and assume power in agriculture. This vacillation between status quo organizing strategies and radical motivations is an important nuance to underscore for understanding how organizations seek "legitimacy" from external stakeholders to acquire resources and political and economic power.

Interdisciplinary researchers have explored the concept of legitimacy in diverse contexts. Mark Suchmann (1995) defines legitimacy as "a generalized perception or assumption that the actions of an entity are desirable, proper, or appropriate within some socially constructed system of norms, values, beliefs, and definitions" (p. 574). In dominant social and political institutions, appeals to "legitimacy" reinforce existing power inequities that align with the status quo (Johnson et al., 2006). Along these lines, William Richard Scott (1995) suggests that legitimacy is more than just a resource, but "a condition reflecting cultural alignment, normative support, or consonance with relevant rules or laws" (p. 45). Pathways to achieving legitimacy are not always linear. Zimmerman and Zeitz (2002) suggest that legitimization strategies typically fall along a continuum of: conformance (adhering to established rules), selection (choosing favorable environments), manipulation (innovating or deviating from past practices), and creation (establishing new social norms, values, or rules). Understanding legitimacy this way helps to illustrate how NWIAA shifted between working within the status quo and taking transformative steps in their quest for external validation and legitimacy.

### *Seeking external validation and legitimacy*

The most salient example of how NWIAA sought legitimacy as an organization was through being recognized by Congress and the Biden administration as a chartered organization. In the United States, organizations with the "chartered" status enjoy a bevy of unique benefits and opportunities, including enhanced prestige, credibility, and visibility (which can attract more donors and grant funding opportunities), influence in policy making and priority consideration for bills, and legal protection against brand misuse (US Government Accountability Office, 2013). For Noreen (US Georgia chapter leader), the legitimacy that came from NWIAA receiving a charter was an important first step for political leaders to take them seriously and for local community members to offer their buy-in.

> Well, it's important because of what we're trying to—the goal is to get the charter, the foundation, so it has to come from a different level. It can't come from the level down here. [Political leaders] have to know. If they don't know, then they can't do anything about it. And then, of course, we have to go through the people on our level to make sure they understand why we're doing that.

Many of the participants shared Noreen's sentiments about the importance of NWIAA securing a congressional charter in their quest for legitimacy. Patience (Ghana chapter leader) also recognized how the prestige of being associated with a US government-chartered organization could lend her indirect benefits such as exposure for her business in Ghana.

> It's something that's going to be of benefit at least to [us as] African women. Someone is going to project African women on that international level. We are going to be heard and more attention is going to be given to us.

Noreen and Patience's narratives draw attention to NWIAA's nonlinear approach to legitimacy. On the one hand, by advocating for new policy with their 4-H pilot program, the women were transformative in that they sought to create new operating practices. Conversely, their approach to food justice aligned with existing economic and political models (e.g., seeking the validation and support of key USDA officials and other food policy actors), and did not seek to fundamentally change or challenge the dominant food system (e.g., modifying *existing* policies, supporting self-sustainable food systems).[2]

Despite direct forms of political disenfranchisement and social and cultural marginalization, NWIAA and its associated women farmers have received varying levels of external recognition and validation for their collective work by key political actors and other power brokers in the United States and globally. For instance, in 2010, the Department of Agriculture recognized NWIAA as an organization in the "Socially Disadvantaged Farmers and Ranchers" resource section on its national website—the only group led by and dedicated to the specific needs of ACB women listed. Tammy discussed the context behind the recognition and the significance of distinguishing the unique needs of ACB women farmers from ACB farmers in general.

> There was nothing out there for women in agriculture. There definitely wasn't anything for Black women. Our organization put Black women on the map and actually gave USDA a reason to start [counting them]. We didn't even exist before the organization started. Yeah. It's crazy. We are still in the shadows if you will, but we didn't exist. [The USDA] couldn't put a number on Black women farmers but they could put a finger on white women farmers. You see how crazy that is? That doesn't even make sense to me…The statistical type data that [Black women] are still kind of lumped in with the Black men as just 'Black farmers'. It's not broke out Black women—and I keep trying to push that issue. We need to get this out here into this data. So therefore the government can see the great need.

The added USDA distinction gave NWIAA a public space for other ACB women to find them and fostered additional collaboration and grant funding opportunities through the Department. Individually, several of the women have received recognition for their community activism and agricultural innovation, which granted them legitimacy and

---

[2] Eric Holt-Giménez and Shattuck (2011) introduced a taxonomy of food system transformation practices built around four axioms, respectively: neoliberal/market-led, reformist/aid-oriented, progressive/empowerment-seeking, and radical/redistribution-enabler, to understand how food movements are aligned in relation to the food regime and their potential to bring about social change.

more opportunities to secure additional funding and build cross-sector partnerships. For example, on March 5, 2024, Noreen (US Georgia chapter leader) had a legislative bill passed on her behalf from the Georgia House of Representatives. "GA HR3141," summarized as "A RESOLUTION recognizing and commending Noreen S Whitehead; and for other purposes" was a formal document recognizing Noreen for her agricultural contributions in the state of Georgia, particularly through her role as Director of the Georgia Women in Agriculture Association (NWIAA) and her efforts to empower women in agriculture, foster youth involvement (such as her AgriTeens youth program) and establish successful farm businesses (Georgia General Assembly, 2024). On that same day, Alexis (US Georgia chapter leader) received the same honor ("GA HR1310"), commending her efforts as a hemp advocate, community organizer, entrepreneur, and project coordinator. Noreen, Alexis, and the chapter members of NWIAA Georgia are also recognized annually by the Georgia state legislature during the "National Women in Agriculture" day held at the Georgia state capitol, in addition to receiving their own commendation from House leaders ("GA HR 1465"; see Figure 4.9).

In Africa, several chapter leaders received recognition from public institutions for their innovations and expertise in things like climate-smart practices, women empowerment, and business leadership. Hawa (Liberia chapter leader) was recently selected as a fellow in the Mandela Washington Fellowship for Young African Leaders program, a US Department of State-sponsored initiative that invites leaders from Sub-Saharan Africa to the United States for academic and leadership training for her pioneering work as founder and executive director of Women in Agriculture for Sustainable Development. Relatedly, Patience (Ghana chapter leader) has received several awards and other recognition from the Ministry of Agriculture in Ghana for her role as co-founder of the Post-harvest Women Foundation, a farmer-based group that empowers women through capacity-building training and climate-smart agriculture practices.

The participants noted not only a rise in external recognition from government institutions but also a significant increase in public interest overall. For example, Alexis (US Georgia chapter member) remarked on the accelerated interest food justice researchers and practitioners

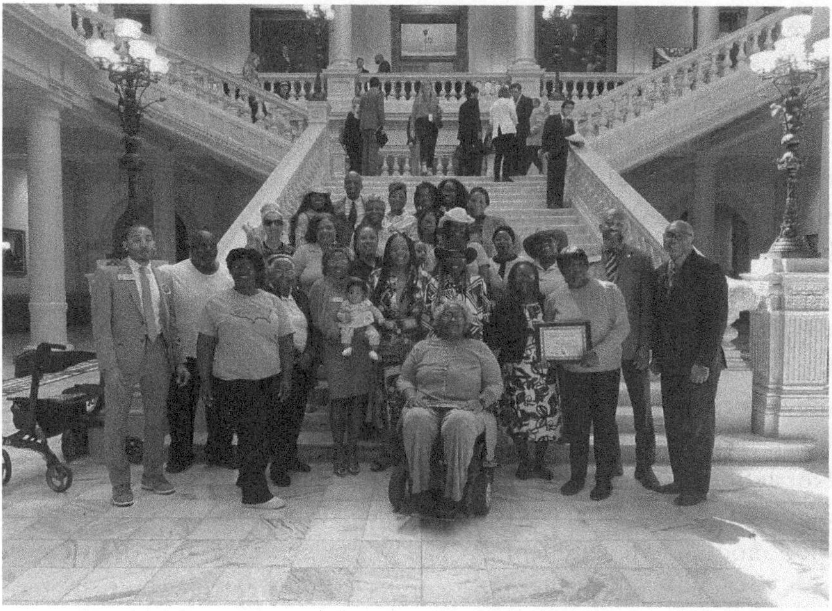

FIGURE 4.9 NWIAA Georgia (GWIAA) receiving recognition from the Georgia State Legislature during "National Women in Agriculture" day at the Georgia State Capitol on March 5, 2024.

Photo by Noreen Whitehead

have taken to studying Black farmer experiences, and how she saw the impact of their research as positively impacting ACB women farmers' perceived legitimacy by top-down stakeholders.

> … there's more interest in Black farmers overall on a national level. This is the third invitation to a university study I've gotten in this month alone, which indicates people feeling the need to highlight our stories, but also give us that verifiable, respected data that we can utilize in funding initiatives.

*Seeking external partnerships*

For the women of NWIAA, being validated and seen as legitimate by political actors was an important first step to developing partnerships with those in power who they perceived could help them get their demands met, regardless of identity or political affiliation. This often included partnering political leaders and external gatekeepers whose voting records and ideological leanings did not support the communities they sought to empower, whom they often asked to speak on their behalf in policy spaces. As a political strategy, NWIAA's "by any means necessary" approach was significant for several reasons. To begin, this strategy was different than other Black food sovereignty movement traditions, which were marked by calls to develop alternative, self-governing food models that existed outside of the dominant food system (Broad, 2016; Smith, 2019). Popular examples such as Fannie Lou Hamer's Freedom Farms Collective, the Black Panther Party's Free Food Program, the Nation of Islam's Muhammad Farms, the North Bolivar County Farm Cooperative, and the Detroit Black Community Food Security Network all pushed for various self-sustaining food models. (McCutcheon, 2013; White, 2011). While the women of NWIAA shared similar motivations and ultimate goals of empowering ACB communities and supporting community food security efforts as the aforementioned examples, their strategy to foster collective agency by working within existing social structures and seeking legitimacy from those in power was a purposeful decision they calculated as their best way to acquire resources given their social position and identities.

Secondly, NWIAA's "by any means necessary approach" was significant in that it complicated notions of Black feminist solidarity. In her influential book *Black Feminist Thought*, sociologist Patricia Hill Collins (2000) outlines a typology for understanding the principles of Black feminism, which include foundational concepts such as the "Matrix of Domination," standpoint epistemology, the importance of solidarity and collective activism, and critiques of respectability politics to highlight how various systems of oppression intersect to uniquely marginalize Black women. As part of an ACB women farming advocacy collective, the participants aligned in principle with many of these axioms in their organizing efforts, though they chose to not always identify *externally* with them because they were seeking legitimacy from external stakeholders within the dominant system and identified such tropes as a way for power brokers to ascribe them group marginalization and not take their embodied knowledge seriously. For example, Keturah (USVI chapter member) and Selena (US South Carolina chapter leader) rejected being labeled a feminist because they saw it as embedded with inferential notions of inferiority and limiting their political agency.

> Because I don't like to think that woman is a minority or something. I don't feel women are. That's not how I really go about my day like, 'Yeah. F the patriarch.' Nah. [laughter] I'm not a feminist or one of those things. But I guess it is a little bit of a reality because that is a view, which makes sense. I see where they're coming from, but it's a little offensive that you think I can't do the work.
>
> (*KETURAH*)

> A lot of times, I'm invited to sit at different tables, and it's because they think I'm going to have a Black voice. And I'm not that person. I have a voice for whoever... So I just said, 'Treat everybody right with kindness and respect and get the job done.' So inviting me because I fit the Black-woman bill, you're not going to get it. But then at the same time, if I say that and you don't like the tone in which I say that, then I become the angry Black woman. So it's like I don't have time to go back and forth and try to explain who I am to people.
>
> (*SELENA*)

Keturah saw being characterized as a feminist by other political leaders in agriculture as laden with preconceived assumptions that she was not capable of doing the same quality of work as men. Relatedly, Selena did not want to be ascribed as the person with the "Black voice" in farm advisory and other externally facing meetings because she interpreted such as a way to pigeon-hole her into assumed philosophical and political orientations that would ultimately limit her capacity to enact agency and secure external resources. Several other participants expressed similar concerns about being ascribed the "Black feminist" label by external power brokers, fearing it could harm their legitimacy and hinder their capacity to secure resources. During my observations, I also noted that when NWIAA leaders were engaging in spaces with non-Black women present (e.g., on Zoom calls, at industry events, etc.), they were intentional to make space for them and identify their group as not exclusively for ACB women. Collectively, the participants' deliberation of such nuanced, microlevel decisions was carefully considered and underscored their acute political dexterity. While at the root of their motivation was a desire to resist dominant structures, their survival required strategic navigation within existing configurations.

In some ways, NWIAA's "by any means necessary" approach has borne success; they have received varying levels of public support for their bill and other programmatic supports from the USDA and other top-down power brokers. However, despite their collective strategy in navigating legitimacy discourses through working *within* existing social structures, racial and gendered forms of capitalism and other inequities generated additional challenges outside of their control that still limited their capacity to develop partnerships with external stakeholders and be recognized as a legitimate group. For example, a chapter leader from one of NWIAA's US South chapters described a situation where she was left out of leadership decisions for plans to develop a regional women's agriculture advocacy collective in her home state by a local group of white women farmers, even though the group initially brought her in to teach them about NWIAA's programs and organizational structure.

> And honestly, since I've started putting out things for National Women in Ag, there has been a group of [white] women that have formed their own [organization] in response to me. And they made a Facebook group, and someone added me to the group, and they were talking about—they wanted to find out ways that female farmers could get grants and what programs were available, and everything that NWIAA [already] does, that I have been, for three years, inviting them to do. And so I got on there and I said, 'Everything's already been established.' I've been asking y'all to join me [at NWIAA] for the last three years. So because you all want to figure it out and reinvent the wheel, I gracefully bow out.

Appropriative actions such as these were not limited to other women, as forms of gendered capitalism also fostered political wedges between ACB men and women farmers. For example, Tammy talked about the process of how ACB women farmers like her often needed to acquire a cosign from a white male farmer to garner attention for funding by many local and national Black male leaders.

> Being an Afro-American female or Black female, you just don't get the respect from Black male leadership, and that's on state or federal level. I've noticed it has to almost be a Caucasian male that gives the okay for them to work with us, for them to take us serious, or to even really communicate with us. Or I've seen where they cut us out of things. Literally, they will take away—we actually won a grant for a million dollars and they cut us down to $400,000 to split between two years . . . However, a Black male organization that doesn't even do a fourth of our work, they have no tangible to show per se [is ultimately awarded grant monies]. Like our organization, you go to the website, you can click and see people, you can get in touch with them by email or phone. It's all right there, unlike others where they just have one or two conferences and they get the exact same money, if not more.

For ACB women farmers, the perceived betrayal of their male counterparts fostered a deeper level of disappointment and something they saw as uniquely detrimental to their capacity to thrive in agriculture. As ACB men and women are often grouped together into one category as a receiving body of resources by policymakers, the unique challenges and barriers experienced by ACB women are often neglected or ignored in such decisions. These inequities are made worse by their self-perceptions of not being taken seriously by ACB male leadership. Related work in political science has documented how intersectional inequities, such as those that emerge from class, gender, and sexuality identities, contribute to a "secondary" marginalization that exacerbates feelings of isolation *within* groups and complicates how collective identities are constructed and mobilized in political struggles (see Brown, 2014; Cohen, 2009). For the women of NWIAA, these collective intersectional challenges forced them to adopt their own *internal* recognition strategies as a protective mechanism and a mobilizing tool.

### Internal Recognition

Along with being recognized for their visions toward transformation and legitimacy from external stakeholders, it is equally essential that resourceful communities internally recognize their own unique cultural and social assets and mobilizing capacity. Given the combined impacts of discursive erasure and racial and gendered capitalism on segmenting collective voice and community capacity, internal recognition is key for resourceful communities to protect cultural legacies and address past and present inequities in agriculture. For NWIAA, these guiding philosophies wove into the threads of its foundational ethos since its nascent stages as an organization.

Tammy laid the seeds to begin an ACB women's farming collective after she noticed the vast absence and lack of representation of women of color across the different agricultural spaces she frequented. As a fourth-generation farmer, she would regularly receive invitations to participate in farm conferences and other events because of her family's legacy status in the community and she saw how women were often not taken seriously for their agricultural expertise and leadership capacities, sometimes being ignored altogether. Driven to make a change, she quit her job as a legal analyst to embark on a new career to empower ACB women farmers. Initially starting out with a small team of legal experts and women farmers, she began by going plot-by-plot in her hometown of Loco, Oklahoma, helping women develop and maintain their land. "We would go out on a Saturday and just break ground for them. We'd have a whole picnic thing and all of us would get together and literally plant a garden or plant blueberries." As Tammy made her local rounds, she was taken aback by the number of women who owned land and had shared family histories in agriculture, but were not able to take full advantage of their lands due to concerns navigating burdensome and exclusionary agricultural policies and communicating their needs and interests to those with access to power—to which her team provided a variety of tools for the women to share experiences and acquire new knowledge. Central to this community-building experience was an emphasis on *sisterhood*. Tammy explained, "we looked at it as a sisterhood because it is a sounding board we have...we get together and we're able to talk about true sister issues being a minority woman."

Participants described *sisterhood* as an important organizing feature of the group and a key component of how they internally recognized each other. Feminist scholar bell hooks (1997) defines sisterhood as a political commitment to solidarity between multicultural women based on shared interests and beliefs. As a resourcefulness strategy, the concept of sisterhood was drawn upon by the participants more regularly than an explicit focus on Black feminist thought, as the former captures the dual exercise of advocating for feminist solidarity while identifying the unique challenges and power disparities experienced by non-white women. Paralleling their *external* recognition approach, employing sisterhood in this way allowed the women to work within existing structures (and not be seen or delegitimized by outsiders as solely a race-based group) while simultaneously building capacity with other ACB women to confer group status "on the basis of common attributes" and position themselves as "a subject of rights and a receiving body for state resources" (Mackinnon & Derickson, 2013, p. 265). For Jadae (US New Jersey chapter leader) and Juhna (US Missouri chapter leader), sisterhood served as a way to foster emotional support.

> Sisterhood means being that shoulder to cry on, to vent your frustrations, to give advice, to give support, to show that you're not alone when you feel like there is absolutely nowhere else to go or no one else to turn to.
>
> (JADAE)

> Sisterhood means when I cry, you cry basically... Just like Brotherhood. Any hood, it's a relationship. When I'm down, I need my sister to pick me up. If my sister down and she's hurting and she's depressed and she's emotional, hey, let's pick each other up. Let's guard. This is therapeutic.
>
> (JUHNA)

Common attributes also include things like shared knowledge, experiences, and struggles (Housel et al., 2018). In this way, other participants described sisterhood as an internal recognition strategy for connecting their cultural knowledge and farming philosophies with other ACB women—which served as both an internal protective mechanism and a strategy for generating group agency.[3] As noted by Tammy, "sisterhood

[3] I discuss how the women described cultural heritage as an "alternative knowledge" resourcefulness strategy in more detail in the next chapter.

was to bring dignity and respect to the minority woman, the Black woman, as a farm operator." For Darceia (US Dallas chapter leader), sisterhood was a way to illuminate the scope of contributions and (hidden) labor of ACB women in agriculture.

> Sisterhood, in the sense that we are women, which is kind of unheard of and not the typical farmer story. I think that that's imperative to know that women can do it, we can do it. Women are farming, women are gutting animals, women are packaging. I think that that's value, but food as medicine is top, and the environmental component that gardening has for our bees and our ecosystem, our soil. We're giving back tenfold. We're taking from the land because we need [but] we're also repairing as we're working.

The participants also described internal recognition processes in terms of making them feel more reputable as agriculturalists. In addition to creating conditions for the women to come together and "take up" space by making them visible to one another and cultivating alternative communication infrastructures, instilling an internal sense of self-respect and reputability was integral for realizing visions of self-determination and shaping "the economic and environmental future in accordance with their desires" (Derickson, 2016, pp. 165–66). Organization theory and behavior researchers have documented the importance of reputability on internal recognition processes (Lee & Abdullah, 2024). For instance, Selena (US North Carolina chapter leader) felt more confident directing her chapter members on where to access resources after NWIAA helped her demystify the process and support her with what she describes as the challenges associated with being a "farmer-by-default."

> [when I work with NWIAA] I feel more farmish. I'm getting out of 'I'm a farmer by default.' I am still a farmer by default. I got to put that disclaimer out there because I don't want everybody to come to me asking myself like, 'I don't know. I have to look it up.' [laughter] I don't know what I'm doing....But yes, [NWIAA has made me feel more reputable as a farmer] because I can say without a doubt, 'okay, yes. You can go through Farm Service Agency and get blah, blah, blah, blah.' But I didn't know that until NWIAA.

Selena characterized herself as a "farmer-by-default" in the sense that she entered into farming due to necessity (rather than by choice or family tradition) after her stepfather passed away shortly after purchasing land with a farm on it. As a self-described "serial entrepreneur," rather than sell the property, she was motivated to find ways to make the land profitable. She reflected: "I knew nothing about farming outside of just the basic gardening and growing flowers with my grandmother and my grandfather when I was a little kid. That's it." For Selena, being a part of NWIAA gave her confidence to maintain her family's land, navigate unfamiliar agricultural spaces, and provide informed guidance to her chapter leaders.

Other participants discussed how NWIAA's name recognition among both grasstops and grassroots leaders gave them an internal sense of confidence to build partnerships and see themselves as reputable in dominant agricultural spaces. Alexis (US Georgia chapter member) and Noreen (US Georgia chapter leader) described their experiences.

> [NWIAA is] a national organization. I, myself, am a sole proprietor. I work in collaboration with a lot of people, but I'm the only staff member. So there's only so much I can do for myself at once. When I'm in the group, they have a lot of different chapters—it's global, so it definitely gives me the opportunity for more exposure and for support of my business.
>
> (*ALEXIS*)

> Because they've been around long enough, and people hear of them. And then just working behind that and just putting in the work and in name. So people know who we are. They know who we are at NRCS. They know who we are at FSA. They know who we are in the community.
>
> (*NOREEN*)

## Conclusion

To deeply explore the unique cultural preservation and political strategies the women employed in their quest to community mobilize, enact policy change, and resist "resilience" discourses, this chapter applied the

*POR* axioms *resources* and *recognition* to the ethnographic data. A specific focus on resources highlighted the participants' unique cultural and social assets and how they developed resistive strategies to subvert discursive and material sites of power (e.g., alternative communication platforms, "weak-tie" partnerships) while an analysis of their external and internal recognition strategies detailed the multiple guardrails and negotiations the women calculated in mainstream political arenas and their internal dialogues to achieve their goals and realize their mobilizing capacity.

*POR's* concept of *resources* builds upon a rich tradition in community-based participatory research of seeking to empower communities to leverage their own assets to address interrelated health and social issues relevant to them. A host of interdisciplinary studies have incorporated similar methodological approaches for developing academic-community partnerships and helping local communities identify and navigate things like storytelling networks, faith-based groups, public spaces (e.g., parks, vacant lots), businesses, and health clinics (see, for example, Lim et al., 2022; Lu et al., 2023). While such models have demonstrated widespread evidence for improving conditions of the populations they are serving, they are often reliant on the academic side of the partnership to leverage skillsets and expertise in "leading the way" for communities to identify their own strengths, resources, and capacities. Further, because many of these interventions are developed through grants and other external funding streams, the ultimate decision-making power in determining solutions often resides in stakeholders outside the community and/or are not fulfilled due to unsustainable capacity and resources. Particularly noteworthy in how the women of NWIAA engaged *resources* was their capacity to largely develop their own asset-mapping techniques without reliance on outside experts. In the context of our academic-community partnership, my collaboration efforts consisted primarily of using my communication training to bring attention to the participants' hidden and erased stories and not co-opt them (in mainstream outlets such as research journals, op-eds, and academic conferences). Since NWIAA had been engaging in this work since 2008, it was clear that they had the requisite expertise and foundational knowledge to understand and develop their own solutions—what they needed was access to mainstream communication platforms to disseminate and normalize their message. Their combined efforts are important to demonstrate the different ways that community expertise and leadership emerge in community based participatory research (CBPR) and asset identifying projects. Building on the belief that local communities are their own best problem solvers, it is often most helpful for academic community partners to "get out of the way" and critically reflect on what they can bring to a particular study context as opposed to assuming leadership in project agendas and outcomes.

The granular analysis of the women's recognition strategies is more than a case study in documenting grassroots political organizing capacity and serves as a helpful heuristic for understanding how marginalized groups navigate intersectional inequities in multilevel public health advocacy efforts. Interdisciplinary CBPR literature has documented processes of community organizing and political advocacy strategies *between* academic and community partner (usually consisting of the academic leveraging their proximity to power and advocating on behalf of the community). However, limited work exists when explaining situations where the community takes the lead in their own advocacy decisions—particularly when they are faced with intersectional race and gender barriers (Chávez et al., 2008; Muhammad et al., 2015). Building on the argument from the previous chapter that access to power alone is not enough to foster equitable social conditions, simply providing access to political power will not ensure that local voices are heard, and change will be enacted. Even though the women were extremely organized and mobilized (i.e., 89 global chapters with transparent documentation of their efforts publicly available) and had access to key levers of power (e.g., the White House, Congress, USDA leadership), their double consciousness reality of constantly having to reflect on their positionality (so as not to appear hyper aggressive or uncivil) and needing co-signs from male power brokers (e.g., republican leaders, Black agrarianists) radically limited their capacity to express full agency when advocating for themselves. As anthropologist Dwight Conquergood (2002) notes, "subordinate people do not have the privilege of explicitness, the luxury of transparency, the presumptive norm of clear and direct communication, free and open debate on a level playing field that the privileged classes take for granted" (p. 146). Due to their multiple marginalized identities as ACB women, they were not able to directly and openly explain the scope of their transformative vision. To bring necessary attention to some of these underexplored visions, the next chapter moves beyond relational contexts to document how the women described alternative "ways of knowing" as applied food justice praxis.

# 5

## "Ensuring Our Yard"

### Alternative Modernities and Futurist Imaginings

THE FIRST TWO EMPIRICAL CHAPTERS in this book grounded the study context and centered the women's voices in how they described relational barriers to securing resources and being taken seriously as agriculturalists, in addition to the level of political strategizing that went into how they sought external and internal recognition. This chapter applies a third concept of politics of resourcefulness (POR), indigenous and folk knowledge, to the ethnographic data to span beyond microlevel realities and observations and document how the women discussed alternative knowledge and transformative visions for food justice and community health. Mackinnon and Derickson (2013) argue that "alternative and shared ways of knowing generated by experiences, practices and perceptions are important spaces of knowledge production about the world," a postulation anthropologist Arturo Escobar (2008) describes as "alternative modernities" (p. 265). Resourceful communities like National Women in Agriculture Association (NWIAA) can draw on these alternative epistemologies as "explanatory frameworks that weave together normative and observational

*Seeds of Sovereignty*. Andrew L. Carter, Oxford University Press. © Oxford University Press (2026).
DOI: 10.1093/9780197789391.003.0005

knowledge, and serve as the guiding framework for shared visions" (Mackinnon & Derickson, 2013, p. 265).

Taking conventional public health norms, practices, and ideological presuppositions of food insecurity cause-effect rationales, measurement tools, and intervention protocols as the status quo, this chapter explores how participants described knowledge around food, land, and agriculture practices. As a resourcefulness strategy, these "alternative modernities" are important for disrupting assumptions that African, Caribbean, and Black (ACB) communities do not contribute meaningfully to food security solutions and are reliant on outside experts who know better. Specifically, the chapter introduces these strategies as they align across people-place connections, cultural heritage, and futurist imaginings.

## People-Place Connections

"Keep left!" These were the final directions I received from the car rental clerk at the Henry E. Rohlson Airport in St. Croix, the United States Virgin Islands (USVI), after she handed me the car keys for my weeklong fieldwork excursion on the island. Said partly in jest, I quickly realized after spending time with the local townspeople that the phrase was less of a formal directive and more of a colloquial salutation to remind mainlanders new to the island of the common convention of driving on the left side of the road. After navigating a few close calls maneuvering out of the airport, I made my way down the highway to meet with Diana (USVI chapter leader). Diana had set up a jam-packed itinerary for me to learn about the local food system in St. Croix and the exciting scope of work happening at her local VI chapter. Shortly after driving through the entrance gates at the Virgin Islands Department of Agriculture (VIDA) headquarters, Diana ushered me into her office to have my pick of different mango varietals and other local fruit from the overflowing box in the corner. The fruit came from the Department's seventy-plus acres of farmland, where local community members could rent plots for personal consumption and learn from the multitude of training and mentoring programs hosted on-site.

As I sat down while she fielded a seemingly endless number of phone calls from local farmers, grant partners, and event planners, I engaged with several members of her team as they checked in to get their assignments for the day. Our conversations ranged in scope from political activist Marcus Garvey's influence on agriculture to the Mango Melee festival that took place on the island the previous day. Once the frenetic pace had settled down, Diana and I exchanged pleasantries and I was then given my assignment: "You will be going with Tafari and Jamal to do farm visits. You will be in the rainforest most of today." Tafari and Jamal were agriculture officers with VIDA tasked with making regular visits to all farm operations on the island to ensure that they were compliant with Department protocols. Following orders, I jumped in the back seat of their Jeep Wrangler as we made our way up the incessantly bumpy and side-winding road into the rainforest. At our first stop, we met a subsistence farmer who owned a small plot of land that she used the acreage to feed her family. In between breaking up a verbal quarrel between her and her neighbor (whose goats she accused of eating her mango trees), she shared detailed stories of the myriad challenges she faced in farming and receiving government support. As she tilled her grounds, I noticed the dozens of rotted mangoes that had fallen off her trees—a common sight across the island due to lack of farm infrastructure.

We visited a total of twelve different farms throughout the course of the week with vast differences in size and scope, ranging from a family using recycled pottery and their front porch to grow vegetables to a Massachusetts transplant, who's recently purchased 100+ acres were so rife with different fruit and vegetable varietals that he needed Tafari and Jamal to explain what they were and how to harvest them. During my course of the visit, one striking observation that immediately garnered my attention was the extent to which the size and scope of individual farms often fell neatly along race and class lines—anytime we visited a white farm operation, it was generally a larger plot of land with more efficient operations, and, conversely, Black-owned farms were smaller, less productive, and on the verge of deterioration. Despite the perceived agricultural abundance on the island, as evidenced by the miles of overgrown moringa, mango, and soursop trees so thick that the sun could not peek through to the rainforest floor, deep-seated inequities in who were able to produce, distribute, and consume food were omnipresent. This observation introduced me to bigger conversations around food and land ownership legacies on the island and in broader global contexts.

Community connections to place formed by agriculture are not politically, economically, and socially neutral, as they are often embedded with histories of settler-colonialism, land theft, dispossession, cultural co-optation, and erasure (Ranta et al., 2022; Williams & Holt-Giménez, 2017). As described in Chapter 2, one of the biggest impacts of racial and gendered capitalism on ACB farming communities—particularly in the USVI and Caribbean—is its role in segmenting resources and unevenly placing capital accumulation within particular spatial scales (e.g., rural, local, regional, global). In the context of resilience policy, Mackinnon and Derickson (2013) argue that this "local-global" divide defines different spatial scales as "arenas for ensuring adaptability in the face of immutable global threats," which ultimately "fosters an internalist conception which locates the sources of resilience as lying within the particular scale in question." (p. 255). Rather than drawing attention to how uneven capital accumulation underpins resilience policy logics, local communities are forced to adapt to a turbulent environment on their own (e.g., addressing land ownership inequities, cultural erasure), which get taken for granted and normalized—assuming what Peck and Tickell (2002) describe as "responsibility without power" (p. 386). From a public health praxis perspective, these resilience logics simultaneously strip local communities of their cultural assets and allow external agents (with more resources and political power) to control decisions pertaining to how resilience solutions are carried out (e.g., metrics used for defining problems/solutions, resource allocation, which expertise "counts").

Diverse interdisciplinary research suggests that land ownership disparities parallel broader inequities in health, socioeconomic status (SES), education, and political power globally (Dachaga & de Vries, 2022; Tseng et al., 2021; Pfeffer & Killewald, 2018; Binder & Binder, 2016), though there is little discussion about the role of land ownership and connection to place as a producer of health injustice and social determinant predicting future outcomes in the context of food insecurity and public health interventions. The women of NWIAA rejected dominant resilience logics that bound them to artificial spatial scales (e.g., zip codes, census tracts, "vulnerable" or "underserved" areas) when discussing how connection to place informed their philosophies to agriculture, public health, and community empowerment, paralleling *POR*'s call to be more scale-specific "in focusing attention on the need to build capacities at community level," in addition to finding ways to bridge these scalar definitions by fostering and maintaining "relational links across space" (Mackinnon & Derickson, 2013, p. 264). A primary mission for the participants was to transcend marginalizing spatial scales imposed upon them by restoring frayed transnational cultural foodways and connections to land across ACB contexts. Alexis (US Georgia chapter leader) described these connections as an inherent characteristic rooted in ACB communities and a guiding heuristic for bridging the local-global gap and bringing disparate women farmers together.

> I feel the shared connection on any land, which is why we are able to have a global division and chapter(s) in Africa. Because some of our same problems here are problems globally. It just looks different, and the narrative might be a little different...That's why I stopped limiting myself. It's like even down to the Black woman experience. There are a lot of things we share in common, but you go to any community, any place you come and unite, it's women who feel a lot of the same feelings. It just looks different or the narrative is different.

The ACB diasporic linkages Alexis makes to land and social problems do important rhetorical work to make transparent the erased ACB agricultural and community connections. Other participants described similar shared linkages in terms of land stewardship and community food security goals. For example, Cheryl (US Alabama chapter leader) saw land as a living organism and something that is sacred and must be protected, which is in opposition to dominant food system logics and policies that take for granted land as a sole means to capital accumulation and inflict widespread environmental degradation (Nesheim, 2015). "The land is sacred. It's a living thing, and we're supposed to be stewards of it. And that's what we try to do, be good stewards." Relatedly, Noreen discussed sharing an ineffable connection and identity with other NWIAA stakeholders regarding commitments to land stewardship and food security, despite not regularly talking to them about such topics.

> Even though I don't talk to them about it, I feel that they share a connection. We all share a connection to the land because that's why we're in this work. We're in the organization trying to feed people. Trying to grow more food. Trying to make sure people are kept on their land. The programming itself is helping to keep people on their land and not get them off of their land. So all of this is a part of that work.

While the participants' shared visions of restoring ACB foodways, agricultural knowledge, and connections to land—if implemented—would indeed have a widespread impact on food security outcomes across food system processes, a multitude of challenges prevented them from realizing such goals. Noreen (US Georgia chapter leader) discussed how policy barriers, such as heirs' property laws, prevented ACB communities from passing down land to future generations, and the steps she was taking with her local chapter members to be better informed on how to address such challenges.

> Some people's land is tied up in heirs property. I've learned about heirs property and how most of the Black land is lost through heir property because they don't know who the land belongs to or somebody sells their portion, which makes somebody come in to get the rest of it. It opens the door. And so now we're making sure everybody has the right documents signed, the deeds signed, the attorneys, those paperworks are correctly documented at the courthouse so nobody could come and take your land away. So those workshops are also being held. And I should be doing a certification course in heirs property.

Interdisciplinary research has similarly documented the devastating impacts of heirs' property laws on land loss among ACB populations (Bailey & Thomson, 2022; Copeland, 2015). Noreen's motivation for bringing awareness to the red tape nuances of heirs' property laws and seeking training certifications to help educate her local community is a growing strategy among ACB food justice activists for preserving ACB land and connection to place (Dyer et al., 2008). This renewed interest has also emerged at the policy level; in 2021, the United States Department of Agriculture (USDA) launched the Heirs' Property Relending Program, an initiative dedicated to BIPOC communities that "provides funds to assist heirs in resolving ownership and succession issues on farmland with multiple owners" (Whitehouse.gov, 2023). Participants also talked about various patriarchal barriers that prevented them from owning and operating land. Betty (Nigeria chapter leader) detailed a story about the challenges she had to overcome in her local city, Port Harcourt by male leaders when trying to own land and the symbolic impact it had on other local women farmers.

> That's a big challenge for women in Nigeria because, when you see a woman that is farming, the land she is using is either a lease or passed to her or owned by her husband or family member. It's difficult to want to actually own a land as a woman. Now I'm talking from experience. At the moment, I am into rice farming. Initially, when I started, I wanted to own my land in the community. It was a 'no' for them. Why would a woman own a land? You have to have someone there that is like a relative that can help you get it. It was a really long fight. I had to lease initially to do my farming. But the second phase of it, I told them, 'You know what? I want to own my own land because I'm making great impact in this community. I'm training the girls on how to do their farming, and I'm bringing different people to the community.' It was a long fight. But eventually, I own my land. So now that's like an eye opener for all the women village. Out of that village, they farm. They have two seasons. They farm all year round. And yet, they don't own a land. So we had to involve some people from the Ministry of Agriculture so these women can own their land if they choose to. So for now, I think we have a few of them that can claim ownership to some lands in the community. I know it's still a long way to go, but that's a win-win for us at the moment.

Black and Caribbean chapter leaders experienced similar patriarchal barriers. Though not legally barred from owning land via de jure legal mandates in some African contexts, they dealt with other challenges that prevented them from owning and maintaining connections to land. Diana (USVI chapter leader) discussed some of the challenges women in the United States and USVI experienced to having success in farming.

> Agriculture is like a male dominated field for the most part. The discriminatory practices when you go to apply for loans and those type of things... historically, [women] were only able to excel in agriculture through their male counterparts. They were the farm wife, you know what I'm saying? They weren't the farmer.

She continued, emphasizing the importance of ACB men and women to work together and how empowering women farmers would ultimately elevate the entire family.

> But it's not about separating the woman from a man. I feel that we do need men and we do need to work together. It's just that we need to provide additional support to women because I know that when a woman succeeds, the whole family succeeds. You're not just doing it for the woman. She has children and they will be inspired by her work or benefit from her work or learn from her work. And that's better education from my perspective.

Diana's commentary corresponds with Tammy's assertion in the previous chapter about the significance for both top-down institutions (e.g., USDA) and Black agrarian communities to differentiate the unique needs of ACB women farmers from ACB farmers in general—both in terms of cultural legacy and the allocation of tangible resources.

## Cultural Heritage

In recent decades, public health scholars and practitioners have drawn increased attention to the multitude of ways that culture impacts health meanings and social practices (Airhihenbuwa, 2007; Sastry et al., 2019). Relatedly, there has been a growing recognition that attending to culture is integral toward "eliminating health disparities, addressing health literacy, and designing and implementing effective public health interventions" (Iwelunmor et al., 2014, p. 20). In the private and nonprofit sectors, organizations such as the Bill and Melinda Gates

Foundation, Feeding America, and the Hunger Project have spearheaded several initiatives that incorporate culture into food and public health interventions (Bill & Melinda Gates Foundation, 2024; Rampersad et al., 2022). Publicly, government programs supported by the National Institutes of Health, Centers for Disease Control and Prevention, Department of Agriculture, and World Health Organization have significantly invested in culture-focused health interventions, particularly through projects aimed at advancing health equity and addressing social determinants of health (Sharma & Sharma, 2024).

While the increased focus on culture as a key metric of health interventions has helped to bring increased awareness to mainstream audiences, many of these initiatives are limited in overall scope and impact (Dutta & Basu, 2011). For example, many public and private culture-focused interventions are rooted in top-down research agendas and incorporate a "culture-as-variable" approach, where culture is reduced to a measurable variable defined, interpreted, and evaluated by experts outside of the community being studied (Ho & Sharf, 2021). Often combined with a "culture as barrier" approach, cultural contexts are seen as encumbrances for "in-need" local communities to adopt the "correct" lifestyle or behavior as defined by cultural out-groups. Even projects that do incorporate the voices and participation of local communities are often done so as a means for engendering cultural authenticity and buy-in, while the ultimate decision-making power remains in the hands of power brokers outside the community (Dutta, 2024; Egid et al., 2021). Moreover, many of the culture-focused public health interventions with larger funding streams often emphasize more fundamental and mechanistic investigations in their program design, as they are often more feasible and easier to demonstrate measurable evaluation outcomes than less studied "edge science" at the community and population levels—whose large scale and scope often requires ample time, resources, and alignment across multiple sectors before tangible impacts emerge (Hoppe et al., 2019; Packalen & Bhattacharya, 2020). Particularly as these interventions situate within the economic and political landscape of capitalism, projects that get selected for funding are often those that promise profitable outcomes rather than cost-prohibitive models that may be more exploratory in nature and lead to less clear cause-and-effect rationales. In the context of food access and insecurity, these approaches often take the form of individual-level change campaigns and do not empower local communities to address structural root causes. More focus is needed on how such interventions authentically and equitably privilege culture as an asset and entry point for exploration as recognized and supported by the communities themselves (Ottemöller et al., 2021).

One potential solution for addressing these challenges is by linking public health and cultural heritage. Heritage scholars define "cultural heritage" as the legacy of attributes of a group or society that are inherited from past generations, maintained in the present, and passed on to future generations (Vecco, 2010). Marilena Vecco describes cultural heritage as comprising three primary components: tangible heritage (physical artifacts such as buildings, monuments, artwork), intangible heritage (traditions, rituals, oral histories, knowledge), and natural heritage (the connection between physical environment and cultural practices). As a strategy for engaging cultural context in local communities, cultural heritage can provide a more comprehensive and holistic account of how such groups make meaning around cultural logics and ultimately lead to more impactful and sustainable outcomes than traditional "culture as variable" and "culture as barrier" approaches. To date, there is scant research detailing the extent to which cultural heritage influences the effectiveness of public health campaigns and intervention designs. Recently, art scholar Bryan Orthel (2022) conducted a systematic review exploring connections between history, heritage, and health within cross-disciplinary literature, and found limited work directly identified a link between these topics.

As an asset-based model, NWIAA represents a case study for exploring how cultural heritage can be used by communities for communities to develop locally created and led upstream solutions. Many of the women discussed heritage as a way for them to preserve, maintain, and pass on histories of ACB cultural foodways to future generations in a way that allowed them to define parameters and take full ownership, in the process reframing entry points for cultural interventions. One way that participants discussed cultural heritage was through recovering past traditions and rituals around food. A primary reason why downstream and midstream public health approaches to food security are not effective is due to their inability to center the deep histories and cultural nuances of the local community and contexts they are targeting. For example, there is a large body of research documenting the pervasive whiteness in many alternative food and healthy eating public health initiatives aimed at ACB and other communities of color, such as farmers markets, community-supported agriculture, and farm internship programs, documenting how these models often romanticize views of agriculture, agrarianism, and food production while limiting participation and interest among such groups (see Guthman, 2011; Marfurt et al., 2023; Levkoe & Offeh-Gyimah, 2020). Noreen (US Georgia chapter leader) detailed how she saw preserving cultural heritage around shared histories as a key first step to restoring cultural foodways and reorienting ACB communities to food and land connections that have been erased over time.

> So that's very important because if we don't have a background, if we don't know where we came from or what we were doing beforehand, we're just lost. We're just roaming around like—that we don't belong anywhere. And we do have a history. We do have a history of taking care of the land. We have a history of taking care of each other. So all of that is mixed up in there. So as we begin to learn how to do things, we find out that, 'Oh, my grandmother used to make this. And she told me about this.' So you can see the signs. But you have to dig deep to find the methods that were used. And those, 'My auntie told me this,' or. There are little things that come out when you're doing things, when we're out in the garden or we're making something. And people remember what they were told when they were younger. And not all of it, but some of it got passed down. But a lot of it did not. A lot of it got lost. And so as you continue to dive in deeper, sometimes you can gain that history back somewhere. That's why a lot of people are going back into their ancestry, trying to find out who they were and who's my great-great-great-great grandfather. Where does it stop? I hadn't done that yet.

Noreen's narrative draws attention to the various challenges ACB communities navigate when trying to restore remnants of their cultural past. Her acknowledgment of how ACB communities' shared history of land stewardship and growing and preparing methods are "mixed up" alongside deeper legacies of erasure and loss highlights complexities in how they rediscover and make transparent these approaches in daily life. Noreen referenced renewed efforts to reconnect ACB farmers to their agricultural heritage and the processes by which ACB communities sought to reclaim land and learn traditional farming methods passed down to them by their ancestors as one way to salvage what they have collectively "lost."

> Because our work, culturally—what should I say? The Black farmers have been left behind in a lot of instances. Lost land. So we're just coming back—I'm glad that I'm able to help those come back to the land in some type of way. Because some have family land. Some had family land. Some want to get land. And they're just trying to find their way to grow again or to learn how to grow the way that their ancestors grew. So a lot of people want to learn how they used to do it back in the day. And they wish they would've paid attention more. They wish they would've listened more, and they would have still had that knowledge. So now they're trying to go find the knowledge wherever they may find it.

From a public health praxis perspective, recovery practices such as "coming back" to the land represent an important upstream, asset-based approach for reenvisioning surface-level, downstream food security interventions that do not engage with the depths of cultural definitions in this way. For ACB communities, another devastating consequence of land loss and cultural erasure is the eradication of diverse locally situated knowledges around nutrition, medicine, and health. Particularly in US contexts (although increasingly global), dominant values that underpin public health nutrition models (e.g., food policy, nutrition guidelines, targeted supplementation programs) are based on models that assume a linear lens to interpreting what "counts" as healthy food (i.e., logics of biomedicine; Hayes-Conroy, 2016; Mol & Law, 2007).[1] Such universalizing frameworks do not account for how broader contextual factors impact on-the-ground realities and interpretations of health nor interrogate the socially constructed nature of scientific

[1] In these models, reductionist Western biomedicine logics reduce bodies to measurable indexes like weight, height, or hemoglobin levels (Mol and Law 2007).

claims more generally (Kimura et al., 2014; McIntosh, 1996). Critical nutrition scholars highlight the ways in which science-based nutrition policy is undergirded by cultural, historical, environmental, and political influences that produce and reify inequities among nondominant groups (see Hite & Carter, 2019; Mackenzie & Murray, 2021). For example, many cultural foods, preparation and production methods, and health perspectives that do not align with the values of dominant nutrition evidence models get hidden, obscured, or constructed as Other—in the process defining such practices as deviant and non-normative (Mayes, 2023; Overend, 2020).

Many of the participants referenced philosophies and practices about food, farming, medicine, and cultural ways of being that aligned outside the purview of dominant evidence models. For example, Atobatele (Nigeria chapter leader) discussed the medicinal value of regional plants in her local community which she learned about via heritage folk knowledge.

> There's this particular plant, I think the English call it jute leaf, or is a Yoruba leaf? We call it a wedu here, and it has a lot of health benefits... do you remember the time of coronavirus? I heard that some scientists from the Arab country, they discovered that particular plant has some healing effects—one of its benefits is that it has a way of killing cancer, and even including the COVID-19 virus. So I think if we are, if I'm able to pass things like that down, I'll be able to tell them that this particular leaf, if you have it, these are its functions, even so you can actually be taking it personally and tell people more about it. And we have a lot of them here. We have a lot of local herbs and vegetables that have great health benefits... we [also] have the pawpaw leaf. Pawpaw helps to reduce and even cure malaria and typhoid, you know, and a lot more of leaves like that, guava leaves, you know, different types of leaves here in our environment. So, yeah, I think that can help. Who knows, who would be able to find cure to some illnesses that are, you know, killing people, and probably even, you know, we'll still have more, more new diseases that will come out. You know, there was a time we didn't know anything about COVID-19, there was nothing about HIV, AIDS. There was really nothing about cancer. You know, these things keep coming up. So with good knowledge about different leaves and their benefits, the future generation

> will be able to help, help have a better world like help, just help in the health sector, or something, sure.

For Atobatele, local plants such as the Yoruba and pawpaw leaf were important cultural heritage tools that she and her local community use (and have used historically) to address health issues. As it pertains to restorative cultural foodways, such practices were even more significant because they centered health and medicine across different levels of the food system (e.g., connecting upstream cultural production/growing practices and knowledges to downstream consumption and availability). However, for many ACB communities, nutrition evidence based in folk knowledges and cultural practices such as these are often framed as Other and "alternatives" by public health knowledge brokers until they are shown to be effective within dominant metrics, despite already being passed down from previous generations as established healing methods (Hassel, 2014). Implicit in Atobatele's narrative is the legitimacy that the scientific community gave her, describing folk practices once they were proven by Western scientific metrics. Coincidentally, recent research has found many traditional Nigerian plants such as the Yoruba leaf and pawpaw to be effective at treating a host of viral diseases (Abubakar et al., 2022); though had it not been for this corroboration by the Western science community, such knowledge would be characterized as inferior and not legitimate by dominant public health nutrition discourses (e.g., nutrition guidelines, certification practices). Further, as traditional knowledge in ACB communities has often been disseminated orally or via other non-written or recorded mechanisms, mainstream cultural logics such as these have further divorced ACB communities from their culturally and historically rooted food practices (Kanu & Ndubusi, 2020; Thompson et al., 2024).

Similarly, Diana (USVI chapter leader) discussed similar cultural discordances in terms of shared communal relationships to food and land that deviate from West-centric practices and logics in the dominant food system.

> ...my culture, growing up in the Caribbean, everybody farms, in your yard. We do plant medicine. You grow up and you know you can use this plant for this. You have menstrual pain, you can go pick this. You have a headache, you go get that. I mean, you want to cook

> something, you go pick up this seasoning. We are ensuring our yard. I have never lived in an apartment in my entire life, you know what I'm saying? So I'm used to—that's part of an extension of ourselves when in some Caribbean families. So it's normal and it's pleasurable to engage in outdoor agriculture related activities.

Diana's assertion of "ensuring our yard" demonstrates how local Black Caribbean communities have found creative ways to resist cultural erasure and advance self-sustainability goals by preserving their cultural food and lifestyle practices. Caribbean food studies scholar Tessa Barry and colleagues (2020) has explored how the region's food system status quo is compromised, in part, due to "patriarchal norms, gender essentialisms, ongoing neo-colonial social relations, and the historical trajectory of the plantation," to which some of the resistive practices noted by Diana become essential for creating sovereign and socially just futures in farming and agriculture (also see Barry & Gahman, 2020; Barry & Gahman, 2021). In addition to protecting legacies inherited from past generations, a key component of cultural heritage involves maintenance in the present. This includes developing material and social strategies for safeguarding cultural and historical resources (Marrero & Mattei, 2022; Fortenberry, 2021). The women of NWIAA sought to manage heritage forms by drawing on culturally centered idioms, reference points, and other contextual knowledge to discursively disrupt dominant racialized tropes in agriculture and keep ACB women motivated to farm. For instance, Tammy and Selena (US North Carolina chapter leader) challenged reductionist farming narratives by describing their fellow ACB women farmers as "divas."

> That's why we called ourselves Agri-Diva, because it just kind of goes with our culture because we like to diva and we like to bling things up. Again, that's our culture. So we wanted to make sure when we reached for those women and spoke to them that they felt that they was an expert. We wanted to make them feel so important but pretty and all the things that was missing. And still to this day, we give roses to our women at our conferences. Even virtually now, we give them we call it virtual pink roses when they do something that they're tearing up, they're doing things. We make them feel real special.
>
> (*TAMMY*)

> There's the advocacy side of farming that's come along with it. And so the Diva In Dirt came about because I was thinking about how that perception of people thinking that a farmer supposed to look like she's rough and rugged and hair not done, nails not done, or no type of self-care when you have to have—so I want to—the Diva In Dirt is to focus on self-care. So no matter what society says you look like, you feel good about who you are and when you look in the mirror. No matter if you see your hair pulled back in a ponytail all over or if it's in curls all the way down your back, however, whatever it is, be comfortable in the skin that you're in.
>
> *(SELENA)*

For Tammy and Selena, referring to ACB women as "divas" was an intentional discursive choice to center shared lived experiences and cultural heritage; the term has historical social and cultural significance as an empowerment symbol among ACB women. In direct opposition to dominant cultural framings of "diva" as a woman who is of high-maintenance, uncontrollable, with a strong attitude and preoccupation with personal appearance, ACB women have reclaimed the term to signify individual autonomy, visibility, and political agency. In the context of agriculture, Tammy and Selena's use of the term makes visible ACB women's cultural heritage in their expressions as farmers, often ignored by both dominant structures in agriculture and traditional Black agrarian communities.

Participants discussed other shared cultural reference points, such as recognizing ACB women as inherent caretakers and nurturers, as integral for managing heritage forms and resisting gendered hierarchies in agriculture. Specifically, participants connected ACB women's unique positionalities and lived experiences in supporting families and communities to broader sustainability discourses around protecting the environment, growing and stewardship practices, and food justice (McCutcheon et al., 2023; Reese & Cooper, 2021). Lucy (Virgin Islands Women in Agriculture Association chapter member), Juhna (US Missouri chapter leader), and Emmanuel (Africa chapter liaison), described these inherent connections by characterizing ACB women farmers as "natural" nurturers.

> I just think in general, just a woman is *naturally nurturing*. Like we're mothers, we can give birth to children. So I think caring for a plant

> is kind of similar to like, caring for a child—not as serious as caring for a child, don't get me wrong. It's like a baby seed you grow, grow into a tall tree, you can watch it grow for its whole life. It's going to be there after you. So I think some women find that *nurturing* to care for a plant like it just feels *natural.*
>
> *(LUCY)*

> Like I said, women, we *nurture*, we *nurture* the kids. We are *nurturers.* We are *natural nurturers* that *nurtures* our youth.
>
> *(JUHNA)*

> One thing that makes the women to actually be so active in farming is the fact that we have noticed that the women are—they are *nurturers.* They are *naturally* gifted to *nurturing.* And part of the ways they *nurture* the children is to provide food for the family. So the women don't want to be at a position where they are helpless without food for the family. So they deliberately get engaged in farming in order to have food for their families.
>
> *(EMMANUEL)*

Arguably, the most vital component to safeguarding cultural heritage is the process of passing it on to future generations. Building on a rich legacy of ACB women, the participants saw this process as integral to protecting cultural foodways and supporting community food security efforts in their local communities; in fact, nearly all referenced working with ACB youth as a primary motivator for them to begin or continue farming. Some of the women discussed being on the verge of giving up agriculture altogether before feeling reconnected through engaging with younger generations. Selena (US North Carolina chapter leader) reflected on one serendipitous moment in her garden when, after growing frustrated from experiencing multiple seasons of poor yields, she remembered her larger purpose for supporting youth, which kept her motivated to continue in the field.

> One day I was out picking blueberries, and it was like the Lord says, 'it's not even about you. It's about these kids' legacy.' And so I was like, let me keep on picking blueberries. And ever since then, my entire attitude has changed or shifted. And then I started realizing the same is true, not just with me, but with other farmers. It's not even about me. It's about being able to feed other people, helping children that

> can't just get food by themselves, learn how to eat, and eat properly and living, just continue to live. And so it has nothing to do with money for me. It has nothing to do with the thank yous, and I need this. It's all to do with our future generation.

The participants' collective motivations to engage in farming as a way to support community food security and safeguard cultural heritage for future generations is a fundamental shift from how we think about food production in the United States and globally, which is done with the primary goal to maximize profits and extract natural and social resources. The women's aim to create generative impact in their own communities through longitudinal strategies (as opposed to short-term aid and charity models popular in public health) introduces new ways to think about interventions with ACB populations that take into account broader structural and historical contexts.

## Futurist Imaginings

In addition to reenvisioning how connection to place and cultural heritage could help restore transnational ACB foodways and protect against community erasure and co-optation, participants also revealed their visions for Black futurist agricultural and public health landscapes. The term "Afrofuturism"[2] was first coined by cultural critic Mark Dery in his 1994 essay "Black to the Future" and gained notoriety as an academic discipline in the mid-1990s and early 2000s—though explorations of its interrelated themes across the arts and sciences date back several decades (Anderson, 2016). Influential Afrofuturist scholars and writers such as Octavia Butler, Kodwo Eshun, Ytasha Womack, Alondra Nelson, Sheree Thomas, and Reynaldo Anderson have advanced perspectives across areas of technology, science fiction, music, literature, art, feminism, and gender, among others. Recently, the popularity of mainstream film and television productions such as Black Panther and Watchmen along with the increased public interest

---

[2] Afrofuturism is a cultural and artistic movement that combines elements of science fiction, technology, and African diaspora culture to imagine alternative futures and explore Black identity and history.

in Black consciousness and experiences emerging from the 2020 social crises has infused new interest in the field among academics and general audiences alike (Griffin & Rossing, 2020). In the context of agriculture, several grassroots activists and community organizations, such as the Institute for Afrofuturist Ecology in New York, New York and Africulture in Fredericksburg, Virginia, have drawn from Afrofuturist perspectives in their approach to regenerative farming, decentralized technologies, and nature-based learning practices.

In pondering futurist imaginings in agriculture, participants shared a multitude of liberatory ideas and innovations toward creating new realities that simultaneously center ACB identities, cultures, and experiences while interrogating dominant narratives of race, technology, and society writ large. Titi's (Nigeria chapter leader) futurist visions included making her state self-sustaining and not reliant on the agendas and support from third sector and development entities. "My vision is to make Ogun State in Nigeria a self-sustaining agricultural state so that I can increase farmers' productivity and income and attain self-sufficiency in food production through modern agricultural practices." Many of the participants detailed specific programs, social impact models, and cultural strategies that connected multiple sectors of agriculture and public health together. Tammy discussed her ideas for fighting food insecurity via developing and sustaining Black futurist agriculture initiatives, which included creating multiple entry points for community members to get involved (see Figures 5.1 and 5.2).

> The primary component, of course, is eradicating food desert issues. That's what we believe in doing, literally, tangibly on the grounds, having these community gardens and people who come in and pick a certain amount... So providing that food system. Providing jobs, creating green jobs. Literally, we hire people to actually maintain the gardens, maintain the record keeping, maintain agribusiness, come in and—we're creating jobs, so economic development. And then they could eventually try to be an entrepreneur or producer of their own. That's the goal, to get them so interested with working with our chapter leaders, and then they branch off and they start doing it themselves and selling back to the grocery stores or what have you or restaurants in their communities.

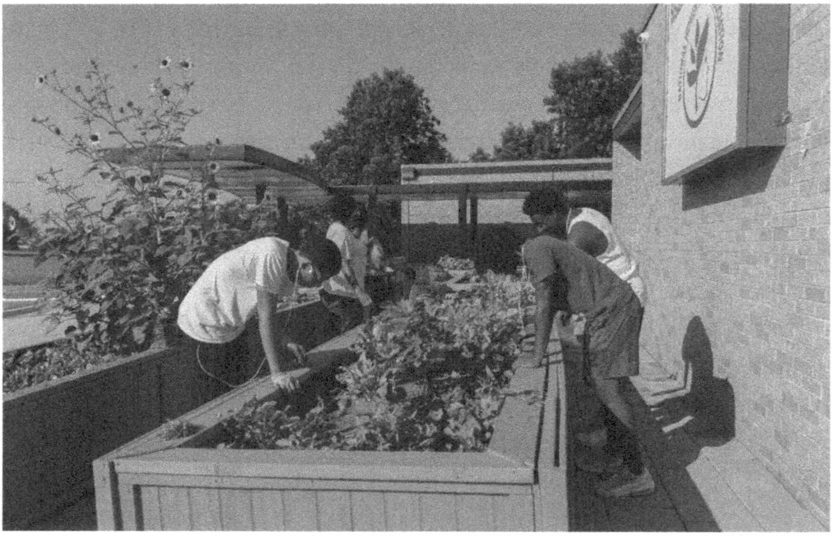

FIGURE 5.1 Youth team leaders working in the raised garden beds at NWIAA Headquarters in Northeast Oklahoma City, Oklahoma.
Photo by NWIAA

Tammy's concept is significant in that it offers an alternative transformative vision for entrepreneurialism in agriculture that is not centered on profit and food as a commodity. Capitalist logics of entrepreneurialism promote minimal government intervention in the economy and favor deregulation, often resulting in weakened policy enforcement and the prioritization of profit over collective best interests, disproportionately impacting low-income communities and communities of color (Ganti, 2014). Conversely, Tammy's (re)framing of entrepreneurialism is done so in the context of communal living and community food security, such that all members of her community can play an active role in supporting the localized food system and become empowered via financial, social, and cultural capital.

Drawing on her background in business and real estate, Crystal (Rhode Island chapter leader) discussed futurist imaginings in terms of connecting generational wealth and community representation to on-the-ground social and public health outcomes. In the excerpt below, she reflected on a conversation she had with a client during a home

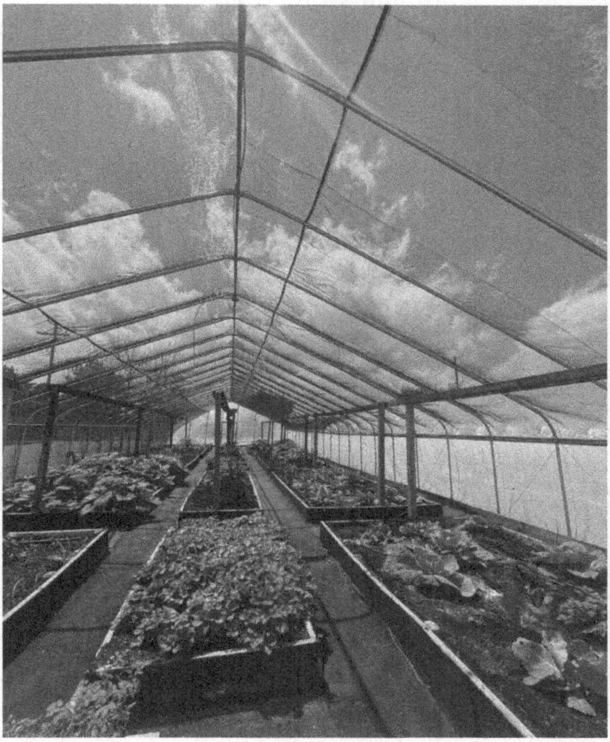

FIGURE 5.2 Community hoophouse at NWIAA headquarters.

Photo by NWIAA

closing about selling to people who look like her, which prompted her to think about the importance of group economics and wealth transfer for upholding ACB community legacies.

> Now, if you get into farming and finance, people are hooking up and connecting to do co-ops, to do Black farming co-ops. We're having the conversation...I just sold a multi-million-dollar house to a 20-year-old. The seller was Black, and she realized—and the girl had an FHA [Federal Housing Administration] loan, one of the worst ones to work with in this market. And she took a $20-something hit. And she said, 'If I sell this house to this young lady, that's legacy.' And I said, 'Huh?' And she's like, 'That's legacy.' She was like, 'Because that extra $25,000 I could put in an account or something for

> my kids.' And she's like, 'The next time they look at [the US Census], the next time they put us all in a group, we're going to be worth more because I sold her a house'.

Nearly all participants offered various visions for new approaches to sharing ACB food rituals, practices, and experiences across local and global ACB communities. Pushing back against dominant narratives and top-down evidence that suggests ACB communities generally do not participate in health promoting food initiatives nor have the capacity to lead such programming due to limited representation and expertise (Carter & Alexander, 2020), the women not only demonstrated their capacity as leaders, but highlighted futurist possibilities for community participation given the proper trust, cultural capital, and sustainable resource channels. Patience (Ghana chapter leader), Selena (North Carolina chapter leader), and Tammy discussed engaging local schools and universities as a futurist approach to food sovereignty.

> Our mission is to go to schools, work with school projects, work with other school organizations, just to project agriculture, make agriculture profitable, make agriculture lucrative, and wanting a girlchild education to improve her literacy rates.
>
> *(PATIENCE)*

> Partnerships as far as just schools. I'm a big, big stickler about our leadership partnering with schools. That's from elementary all the way up to high school. And we're highly partnered because I know how important it is that this stuff getting to our children's soul, if you will, at an early age...And it could be land grant or just an agriculture college, because, again, you have agriculture colleges, junior colleges that are not land grants. So long as they have some type of agriculture or science aspect to it, deal with environment or things like that, I'm okay with that.
>
> *(TAMMY)*

> I'm partnering with the schools...we're going to the school, afterschool programs, in all the elementary schools, teaching them agriculture. We've put up tower gardens in two schools, and we just got a grant through Piedmont Community College for three more gardens. So now all of the elementary schools will have those tower

> gardens, and I'll be maintaining and monitoring those gardens. I'm on the Education Collaborative, and we are making sure that the youth are supported in education.
>
> *(SELENA)*

The women's strategies for working with schools as an entry point toward addressing ACB youth health literacy and food insecurity are not uniquely innovative per se—there is ample interdisciplinary scholarship demonstrating the impact and cultural relevance of local food producers partnering with local schools to address food system-related inequities (Bagdonis et al., 2009; Seguin et al., 2017)—however, their positionality as ACB women makes their approach distinctive. Many Afrofuturist writers have advanced notions of the philosophy as a radical form of science fiction, utopian, otherworldly experience that exists outside of the realms of day-to-day life, however for ACB women farmers, whose mere existence has largely been erased and forgotten by dominant society, the tangible and applied examples shared by Patience, Selena, and Tammy serve as radical innovations and reenvisionings on their own accord.

NWIAA's multigenerational collective of women brings a wealth of lived experiences, cultural assets, knowledge, and expertise to Black futurist thought provocation. Many of the participants were introduced to agriculture as a second career later in life after seeing the impact that growing food had on their local communities. Bridget Pettis (Arizona chapter leader) and Ruthie Bolton (Mississippi chapter leader) came to farming after hall of fame careers in the Women's National Basketball Association (WNBA) and saw the field as fertile ground for fostering ACB futurist visions around food activism. As the premier professional women's basketball league in the United States, the WNBA reported viewership of over 36 million unique total viewers across all national networks and revenue generating approximately $200 million in 2023 (Hague, 2023). As the sport grows in global popularity, those numbers are forecasted to continue rising (Wile, 2024). Importantly, the league has a rich legacy of being on the front lines of fighting for gender and racial equality (Everbach et al., 2022; Williams, 2022). Recently, in 2020, league leadership offered its support when players from the

Atlanta Dream advocated for the Black Lives Matter movement by wearing t-shirts with the phrase affixed on them to games, which led to a clash with team co-owner and Georgia Senator Kelly Loeffler, ultimately resulting in her selling her stake in the team (Deb, 2020). Bridget and Ruthie have built on the WNBA's legacy of transformative justice to bring perspectives about food sovereignty to their fellow players in the league and the general public alike. Bridget reflected on the time when she first brought up the idea of growing food and agriculture to her sister's teammates in the league.

> It was definitely unique. When I brought it to the—my sister is in the WNBA. They were like, 'What?' It just seemed like it was so far-fetched. But at the same time, everybody, and I mean every player that I've talked to, they all wanted their own garden. And they all wanted to learn how to do it. And even this spring, I'm going to be doing a workshop with former [WNBA] players on how to build their own gardens and getting them back out in nature. I just think that the ways of the world kind of led us back in our houses. And this was one of those pieces as a woman. And a lot of the players have children. They want healthy children. And this makes sense. They see the type of food that's in our system today in our environment. And we're eating a lot of fake food. And they know it. We know it.

Recently, Bridget has catapulted to be one of the leaders in food justice activism among women athletes in the United States. In 2024, the WNBA held its annual All-Star Game in her residence of Phoenix, Arizona. During the days leading up to the game, her Bridget Pettis Foundation hosted the "Beyond the Game: Uniting from Arizona to Africa" fundraiser, which was a week-long affair of different activities that brought together members from the local Phoenix community and dignitaries from the WNBA and various other entertainment sectors. One of the featured events during the week of activities was the "Taste of the Garden: Farm Experience," which included a culturally relevant farmers market, local garden tour, and drum circle; the event was meant to bring food justice awareness to the local Phoenix community and promote global women empowerment. In addition, Bridget runs her All-Star Skilled Basketball Camp in East Chicago, Illinois and Phoenix, which is a hybrid program that teaches youth basketball skills and introduces them to farming and sustainable agriculture practices at a young age. Bridget's collective efforts reflect a growing futurist vision for introducing young ACB women to farming and agriculture.

Similarly, Ruthie built upon this futurist vision connecting youth basketball with farming education as a way to share ACB food rituals, practices, and experiences across local and global ACB communities. Growing up on a farm in Mississippi, she learned from a young age the individual health and community benefits of agriculture. Throughout her playing career, she regularly farmed and grew her own food, crediting her diet and way of life for much of her success.

> One thing about the farm and the exercise and being out in the field, I know it contributed to my success. I made sure that when I was playing, that I kept my protein up, and I ate my, you know, my beans and my greens and—I just loved my vegetables... so without a doubt, just the things and the way I grew up and what I ate and what I continue to eat, because it was instilled in me.

Today Ruthie hosts various basketball camps that infuse on-the-court skill training with farming and agriculture education. During one of our conversations, she reflected on the reaction her campers often have when they are first exposed to farming (see Figure 5.3).

> And we actually did a clinic, I want to say, last year, the year before, a basketball clinic. And we had, at the break, they were learning about farming and learning about planting. And I thought the kids were gonna think we were crazy. Like, why are you bringing this to a basketball clinic? They were so intrigued. Like they were so curious. Like, how can you put this in the ground, dirt, and then this comes out of it? And so, just really to be able to see the hands-on, and seeing what it does for the youth, it's so powerful!

Participants also discussed futurist visions in finding new and sustainable ways to expose and train ACB youth in agricultural technology. Opposite of dominant approaches to ag tech, which reify existing inequities in agriculture via "efficiency" discourses that

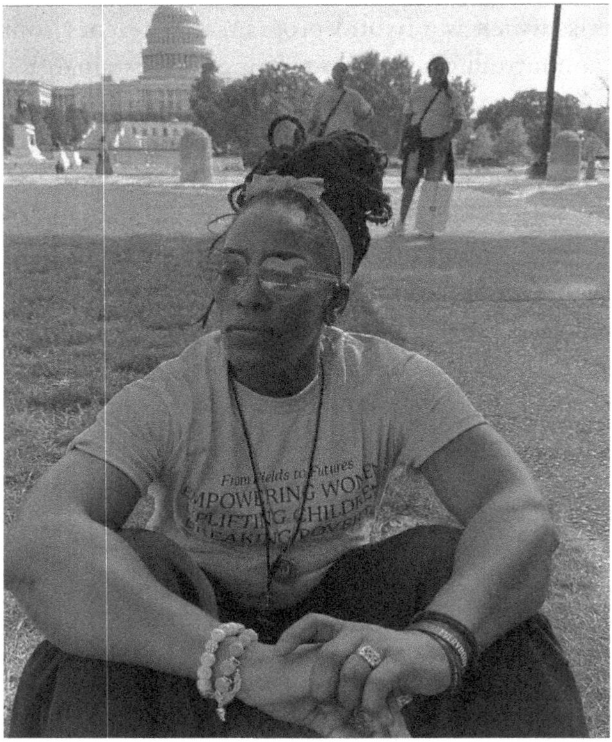

**FIGURE 5.3** Ruthie Bolton attending the NWIAA "Equity and Inclusion" protest in Washington, D.C. on September 21, 2023.

Photo by NWIAA

produce and reproduce land displacement and consolidation, labor exploitation, environmental racism, and knowledge erasure (Carcamo et al., 2023; Rotz et al., 2019; Galaz et al., 2021), the participants offered new ways to think about technology that centers and protects ACB knowledge and cultural contexts, while still emphasizing benefits of increased productivity, shared decision making, and sustainability. Darceia (Dallas chapter leader) discussed her vision for providing ACB youth access to drones in agriculture via culturally relevant channels such as the Black church.

> I'm bridging that gap trying to pitch right now for drones and robots so that it can be more technology in it, so that they can check the soil

> a different way, and then I can talk to you about what you should look for. But first, I want to get you out there and see how this technology works. And I think that that's also another cool thing that can happen in Sunday school at the church.

Historically, the Black church has held a place of spiritual, political, economic, social, and cultural significance and a conduit for engaging in political activism and youth education, and health initiatives (Carter-Edwards et al., 2012; McDaniel, 2009). Relatedly, Tammy and Emmanuel (Africa chapter liaison) discussed futurist visions for introducing agricultural technology to ACB youth via a local community-supported curriculum that built upon ACB knowledge and cultural contexts.

> And right now, we also have a proposal where we can open model modular farms in secondary schools. That model modular farms will enable us to teach young people agriculture using model technology in line with their curriculum—a curriculum that the secondary school education board have set in place. We can be able to connect with that curriculum but employ new teaching methods. So these are some of the visions we have for the African chapters.
>
> *(EMMANUEL)*

> I would envision it here at headquarters that we would have it as an actual training tech school. The goal is to have where we could pay scholarship six people every six months to come through our program that would be able to grow food, sell food, but then also be going to an apprentice program to train six more, and keep that going. So therefore, we're producing more farmers, literally and figuratively.
>
> *(TAMMY)*

Paralleling the participants' perspectives and technology as a common theme in the Afrofuturism literature, scholars and activists such as A. Breeze Harper (2009; 2011) and a growing list of popular writers, bloggers, and podcasters have similarly explored Afrofuturist concepts in the context of things like decolonization, veganism, and moral consumption practices. These corpora of diverse ideas contribute new ways of thinking about how Black futurist perspectives can be incorporated into existing agricultural and public health landscapes.

## Conclusion

This chapter explored how the participants described indigenous and folk knowledge with reference to their transformative food justice and community health visions. By documenting how they advanced "alternative and shared ways of knowing" in the context of people-place connections, cultural heritage, and futurist imaginings, the findings introduce potential frameworks for disrupting dominant public health organizing logics and radically reenvisioning local and global food systems.

Some of the participants described processes of "getting back to the land" as a way to preserve cultural heritage and recover past traditions and rituals around food. Similar strategies have been popularized recently by other food sovereignty scholars and activists, particularly in urban agricultural contexts,[3] as a meaningful grassroots approach for (re)connecting communities to land and culture (Colson-Fearon & Versey, 2022).

In mainstream US contexts, many of these philosophies have garnered attention, building on the popularity of various back-to-the-land and counter-culture activism movements of the late 1960s and early 1970s. Particularly in places like Northern California, activist projects such as the People's Park in Berkeley and the Diggers (an anarchist community action group based in San Francisco's Haight-Ashbury district) set the landscape for various alternative food projects in the decades to follow (Alkon, 2012). These early movements were rooted in a collective self-sufficiency and saw the act of growing food and pastoral living as a form of resistance by linking environmentalism to the nonhierarchical, decentralized organizational forms favored by the oppositional politics of the New Left activists and the counterculture (Alkon, 2012; Guthman, 2003). Despite their lofty democratic ambitions, these movements were largely exclusive and centered a white identity politics

[3] Urban agriculture includes the cultivation, processing, and distribution of agricultural products (food or non-food) in urban and suburban areas (USDA, n.d.)

that appropriated from non-white traditions, especially those of Native American groups, that were viewed as premodern models for a post-modern future (Bowdler, 2021). In many ways, the back-to-the-land movements of the 1960s and 1970s served the racial and class interests of its participants and, despite its egalitarian ethos, ended up reinforcing dominant cultural trends (e.g., post-World War II consumerism, emphasis on "politics of the personal," and the settler-colonial appropriation of Native culture (Bowdler, 2021).

This context is important to note when discussing how ACB communities think about ways to get "back to the land." To begin, dominant "counter-culture" narratives are most remembered and cited in today's mainstream discourse (Rasmussen, 2024). These accounts have largely centered on white experiences in these stories and erased the perspectives and unique cultural histories of non-white groups in these contexts. At the same time, for some ACB communities, discussions about "getting back to the land" requires them to relive past traumas of slavery, sharecropping, and peonage systems—creating a fracture in how diverse ACB communities think about resourcefulness and reparations this way.

Recapturing historical "back to the land" narratives can serve as a praxis-oriented, upstream model for realizing transformative food and public health visions. However, it is essential that ACB communities themselves lead these initiatives to make sure they authentically and meaningfully address cultural barriers of past trauma and violence and ensure that leadership and agendas are not co-opted and overtaken by romanticized narratives outside of their communities.

The collective narratives featured in this chapter serve as foundational anchors for the next steps ahead. As an all-encompassing site of political and economic power, the dominant food system has been able to exist protected and largely unchecked as a governing model due to entrenched agricultural policies and top-down logics (e.g., beliefs that our current food system is the most efficient and capable of feeding the most people) which get framed as universal. To subvert the dominant system will require the infusion of multiple alternative perspectives that shine a light on the potentialities for change.

# 6

# Conclusion

I BEGAN THIS BOOK BY retelling a brief vignette of Black Wall Street (BWS) and the Tulsa Race Massacre of 1921 to highlight how the unique social circumstances and cultural context of the time offer a blueprint toward the possibilities of Black sovereignty in the twenty-first century—introducing the National Women in Agriculture Association (NWIAA) as the evolution of a new global BWS movement. In the years directly following the massacre, the residents of Greenwood rebuilt much of the original neighborhood. The move was largely a resistive act in response to the unfair zoning laws enacted by racist city leaders following the massacre mandating that Greenwood's former residents move further north, away from valued land in the downtown area and railroad access to free up space for local white businesses to develop. Ultimately, Greenwood's residents won a lawsuit that stopped the city from preventing former property owners from rebuilding their homes and businesses. Though not quite the bustling city center it once was prior to its destruction, the rebuilding of the Greenwood District was symbolic in that it represented the collective resilience of its local Black residents to come together and overcome adversity.

Revisionist historical accounts often emphasize this specific aspect of the story, highlighting the neighborhood's forty-five years of prosperity

*Seeds of Sovereignty*. Andrew L. Carter, Oxford University Press. © Oxford University Press (2026).
DOI: 10.1093/9780197789391.003.0006

after the massacre. However, a frequently overlooked part of Greenwood's rebuilding narrative is that the reconstructed community would eventually be demolished again—this time through more indirect and politically nuanced ways. Following the brief period of economic boom, myriad urban renewal projects—such as the Federal Highway Acts of 1965 and 1968 that built a network of highways that directly intersected the neighborhood—were spearheaded in alignment with broader trends across the United States that dismantled Greenwood's infrastructure and displaced local residents. The renewal efforts not only stripped the district of its material space but also eroded its cultural significance and historical legacy—an interminable loss still felt today by its residents.

Appeals to resilience are a common thread in both the revisionist account of Greenwood's rebuilding and dominant narratives in today's public health and agriculture landscape. Similar to how the residents of Greenwood were celebrated for their ability to remain resilient in the face of direct violence, Black farmers and their communities are routinely implored to adopt similar coping strategies in the face of adverse circumstances such as inequitable food access, climate change, and discriminatory policy legislation. Of course, these discourses do not account for the structural conditions that birthed the realities for these groups to remain "resilient" in the first place, nor the repeated insults that deem this characteristic a pervasive necessity. Rather, it may be eminent domain and urban renewal processes, United States Department of Agriculture (USDA) racial discrimination, or prohibitive land ownership laws, any legitimate discussions on social justice and transformative change must move past symbolic, microlevel solutions to address structural root causes.

Fundamentally, *Seeds of Sovereignty* is a transformative text, offering new entry points for thinking about how we organize our food and public health systems and whose voice leads those discussions. Through this manuscript, I examined the historical lived experiences, political voice, and locally situated knowledge of African, Caribbean, and Black (ACB) women farmers and their capacity to support food security, preserve cultural heritage, mobilize locally and globally, and restore frayed cultural foodways. Drawing on the theoretical tenets of *POR* (Mackinnon & Derickson, 2013) and grounded in ethnographic and participatory action research, I documented the women of NWIAA's political organizing strategies as a case study for exploring how ACB women farmers navigate structural and relational inequities, generate and preserve social and cultural resources, and envision transformative futures for food justice and community health. Importantly, I argued that the women's philosophical approach to growing and distributing food provides an innovative model for rethinking asset-based, upstream public health interventions, particularly among low-income communities and communities of color.

In this concluding chapter, I outline the book's key empirical and theoretical contributions and discuss broader implications and takeaways for scholars and practitioners advancing this work across different sectors and subfields. I also reflect on the future possibilities of food system organizing and public health praxis against the backdrop of one of the most polarizing social and political landscapes in recent memory.

## Central Contributions of the Book

*Seeds of Sovereignty* makes several significant contributions to existing literature and broader public conversations about public health, agriculture, and strategies for social justice and community organizing. Today's food system is a far cry from what it once was, even seventy-five years ago. In the United States, visions of small-scale, family-owned, diversified, and independent farms have been replaced by the predominance of multinational corporations controlling vast and complex agricultural networks that prioritize efficiency, profit, and mass production. In Africa and parts of the Caribbean, romanticized notions of community farming and local trade have been supplanted by export-driven monoculture crops and billion-dollar seed conglomerates that hold monopolies over where and how food is produced. Complicit in this structural shift is the global public, who have largely consented to this model as the best (and only) way to organize our food system in a way to meet the demands of a growing global (and increasingly food-insecure) populous. This complicity gets reinforced regularly through policy decisions and the everyday stories that we tell about nutrition, food access, and health. However, largely obscured in this consent are the myriad un[in]tended public health, environmental, and social risks that, in many ways, have created more problems than solutions.

The women's stories featured in this book ring the alarm that our current way of structuring the food system is neither the *best*—nor *only*—way to address these multifarious challenges. As noted in the introduction, their narratives do not exist in isolation and are part of a larger chorus of ACB women farmers who have similarly drawn attention to these concerns, though their collective voices have been systematically segmented and erased from mainstream consciousness. One key contribution of *Seeds of Sovereignty*, then, is to provide a platform for ACB women farmers' political voice to infiltrate the mainstream. Their unique positionality brings a wealth of insight into the combined strengths and challenges of community-based political organizing and why dominant cause-and-effect rationales about ACB health disparities and food access are both wrong and dangerous.

As I have argued in this text, one of the largest consequences of Black women farmers' erasure is the combined deleterious impacts of fractured collective memory on ACB transnational foodways. From early periods of colonization, through slavery, to the myriad challenges impacting ACB communities in the contemporary food system, ACB women farmers have remained on the front lines of protecting cultural foodways and engaging community food security efforts, though their rapid extinction threatens to permanently impact global communities writ large. Given ACB women's capacity to uphold their communities throughout history in the face of adversity, it is perhaps unsurprising then that they are the torch bearers of this new diasporic movement for food sovereignty.

Scholarly discussions about reconnecting ACB diasporic communities are not new. Dating back to the early twentieth century, a host of Pan-African activists and writers such as W. E. B. Du Bois, Marcus Garvey, George Padmore, and Frantz Fanon were some of the first individuals to bring this school of thought to the mainstream. In the context of food and agriculture, there is a growing chorus of researchers and writers, such as Priscilla McCutcheon, Shakara Tyler, and Jahi-Johnson Chappell, who have theorized these principles to engage a diverse group of audiences. NWIAA is one of the first community-based, women-led organizations to apply these philosophies in real, on-the-ground contexts. Admittedly, the women are in the nascent stages of this level of organizing and the longitudinal impact of their work is far from evidentiary; however, their mere courage and innovation to think about community-grounded solutions in this way represent an important first step toward the development of more permanent ones. Early successes, such as gaining the attention of White House officials and other global agricultural leaders, serve as a formative blueprint to creating transformative and sustainable public health change.

Building on this innovation, the research from this book is situated alongside a limited but growing repository of work applying politics of resourcefulness (*POR*) to food systems transformation in the context of Black farming communities (see Lindemann et al., 2022; Ranganathan & Bratman, 2021). Theoretically, *Seeds of Sovereignty* is one of the first applications of the framework to study ACB women farmer experiences specifically, introducing an intersectional lens for envisioning resourcefulness strategies. The women's stories featured in this text demonstrated how their social identities (particularly race, gender, and class identities) were central to interpreting theoretical findings. This text presents insightful perspectives for researchers seeking to apply *POR* in food systems related to this specific population.

## Seeding Change: Takeaways for Practitioners and Scholars in Public Health, Agriculture, and Beyond

The findings presented in this book document the micro and macrolevel strategies of ACB women farmers to mobilize resources, navigate political structures, and protect knowledge as a means for preserving cultural foodways and addressing community food security. Though the results are reflective of a single case study, there are many important takeaways that can be applied to various other contexts and audiences. In this section, I explore broader lessons learned for practitioners and scholars engaging in food justice work across fields of public health, agriculture, and beyond.

The primary audience for this book is public health. Given the field's emphasis on population-level outcomes, community well-being, and various applied and praxis-oriented approaches, there is great potential for practitioners and institutions to incorporate some of the women's philosophies and referenced strategies into intervention and policy design. As the foundation of food systems, agriculture has immediate public health impacts on things like community nutrition outcomes, food availability, and overall economic stability. However, as I have argued in previous chapters, most public health initiatives do not make clear links to agriculture production and distribution processes, often incorporating them (if at all) as ancillary components of a larger intervention. In these cases, agriculture is theorized through downstream, consumer-based solutions such as Supplemental Nutrition Assistance Program (SNAP) incentives at farmers' markets or food voucher programs, missing the opportunity to more directly foster multi-sector alignment.

In this vein, one important takeaway is for public health practitioners to identify these links and make them more salient. Of course, combining agriculture and public health in this way should not be done so from the confines of our current food system—the one responsible for worsening inequities in land ownership and scale of farm operations, the exacerbation of water pollution through nutrient runoff, the degradation of vital soil resources, the emission of greenhouse gases that accelerate climate change, increased pesticide exposure and community food insecurity rates, among a host of other problems (Anderson, 2021; D'Odorico et al., 2019; Neff et al., 2009).

The women's narratives offer new entry points for how practitioners might initiate this work. For example, their particular focus on children as a priority population draws attention to the importance of creating sustainable and culture-centered programming that connects youth to agriculture and public health. Structural interventions like NWIAA's congressional proposal to create specific 4-H programs for Black youth in agriculture and other strategies toward engaging ACB youth, such as promoting youth entrepreneurialism as "communal living," supporting ACB women leadership roles in school public health and farming initiatives, and introducing farming to youth in community-invested programs such as basketball clinics and the Black church offer starting points for practitioners and institutions to develop more meaningful and effective interventions. To be clear, introducing youth to farming and healthy-eating practices is not a novel public health insight on its own accord per se, as there exists a wide range of initiatives and campaigns that draw on these strategies, such as farm-to-school and nutrition education programs, urban farming initiatives, community and school "teaching" gardens, among others (Hume et al., 2022; Mishra et al., 2022). However, many of these frameworks are predicated on the securing of grants and other external funding, creating vast inequities in which communities have the capacity to advocate for these programs and keep them sustainable (Allen & Guthman, 2006; Herlitz et al., 2020). Further, these types of programs, which are regularly positioned to help "under resourced" or "communities-in-need," do not often resonate with their "targeted" populations, as they fail to engage with broader discussions around cultural meanings of food and alternative/indigenous agriculture and farming practices and are not led by leaders in the community (Kolavalli, 2020; Slocum, 2007). By centering community expertise and directly advocating for state resources, NWIAA offers a more sustainable and culturally relevant model that can more equitably impact ACB communities.

Relatedly, the participant's recognition that engaging children with agricultural concepts and practices during formative years can have a cascading effect on their knowledge, attitudes, and behaviors related to agriculture, health, and sustainability as they progress through life stages brings attention to thinking about agriculture from a life course perspective. The life course model is an organizing framework for explaining health and disease across populations and over time and has been used to study a range of phenomena, including adverse childhood experiences, maternal health, chronic disease prevention, environmental health, and the social determinants of health (see Clifford et al., 2016; Hilal & Brayne, 2022)—though there is scant research exploring how it applies specifically to histories of food production and farming. The limited existing work in this area tangentially addresses phenomena such as food choices and nutrition from a downstream perspective (see Devine, 2005; Herman et al., 2014). The women's approach to addressing food insecurity by engaging broader tenets of the food system (e.g., farming education, food production and distribution, land stewardship) represents a novel strategy for public health practitioners to think about ecological approaches and multi-sector engagement.

These collective entry points also offer insights into public health pedagogical practices. For example, schools and departments of public health that teach different aspects of the food system can (and should) incorporate some of these perspectives into their curriculum design, such as the role of cultural foodways in determining on-the-ground experiences of food insecurity and access and how land allocation histories and (re)distribution can be explored as a form of critical public health praxis. Many existing public health degree programs that offer studies in food and health from a community or population perspective often emphasize consumer-level components such as nutrition education and health promotion efforts aimed at guiding "targeted" communities down the correct pathway to "eating healthy" and "making the right choices." For programs that do explore upstream-level determinants such as food access and environment, there remains a missing link when it comes to critically interrogating (and centering) deep histories of subjugation and erasure at the level of food production and how those contexts influence everyday realities for communities in their curriculum.

*Seeds of Sovereignty* also offers a set of unique, yet interrelated takeaways for academic and practitioner audiences in the fields of farming and agriculture. The most salient takeaway from the book encourages relevant stakeholders to move past the current status quo of how we organize our food system and seek out opportunities to radically reenvision what is possible. Most likely, this will require audiences to suspend dominant cultural logics associated with the existing corporate agribusiness model, which comes pre-laden with a set of assumptions about how society makes sense of food scarcity, cost, nutrition, and healthy eating narratives. For example, common conventions in agriculture rhetorically construct a false binary that pits small-scale, "alternative" versus "conventional" large-scale/agribusiness practices in opposition to one another (Sumberg & Giller, 2022). While small-scale models are often promoted as useful approaches for supporting local economies, empowering grassroots communities, and developing democratic local food systems, critics argue these approaches are unsustainable for meeting the demands of the global food system and position the large-scale corporate agribusiness model as the best way to maximize efficiency and meet these needs. However, this constructed binary reifies several falsehoods. To begin, the dominant system is *not* efficient, as approximately thirty to forty percent of the food produced in the conventional food system is wasted every year, contributing to eight to ten percent of global greenhouse gas emissions (Food and Agriculture Organization of the United Nations, 2011). Additionally, this dichotomy obscures the myriad other approaches to food systems organizing that exist within and across these poles that traverse social sectors, economic models, political philosophies, and cultural logics. A sample of other organizing philosophies from across the globe, including sustainable farming, policy models, and land reform movements in geopolitically diverse regions such as the European Union, South America, and Japan (Kondo et al., 2024; Maysels et al., 2023) help to decenter the dominant model as universal and levy alternatives.

This artificial binary also constructs corporate agribusiness as the most scale-specific model for feeding the most people, although the extent to which that happens is unequal. A host of interdisciplinary literature has documented the myriad ways low-income communities and communities of color are disproportionately tied to the negative impacts of the dominant food system (e.g., diet-related diseases, increased pesticide, genetically modified organisms (GMO), and pollution exposure), as they have limited agency to choose what food to eat and where to purchase it from (Conrad & Zuckerman, 2020; Odoms-Young & Bruce, 2018). High resource communities, conversely, can more easily escape these deleterious social, public health, and environmental consequences, and, in many instances, choose to sidestep the dominant system altogether by having the political and economic agency to support alternative models (e.g., organic food stores, community-supported agriculture programs, farmers markets) that prioritize things like small-scale, local, and community-led and supported food production, environmental sustainability, and high levels of consumer awareness (e.g., where and how their food is grown, fair trade and other ethical sourcing practices, "slow," local, and other alternative philosophies around growing and consuming food; see Alkon & Guthman, 2017). Notably, rooted in many of these alternative models are the same philosophies that the women of NWIAA champion in their advocacy—though their approach has broader application and more potential to liberate low-resourced communities in the process. Since its inception in 2008, NWIAA has continuously heard from political leaders and the public that its model, despite being lauded for its ambitiousness, is not financially nor logistically sustainable at scale. However, if we are to suspend dominant cultural and capitalist logics associated with the existing corporate agribusiness model and seek out opportunities to radically reenvision what is possible, the more salient focus should not revolve around how models such as these are *not* possible, but rather, how do we organize resources and develop policies for the grassroots visions such as the women of NWIAA to "scale up" and meet the critical need of diverse global communities?

Finally, the book offers several critical insights for social justice scholars and practitioners, particularly those interested in grassroots organizing, intersectional advocacy, and the complex interplay between local and global justice efforts. Importantly, the book adds new dimensions to conversations on how marginalized communities engage in multi-sector collaboration and advocacy. The women's approach to securing sustainable funding by combining grassroots community organizing and grasstops outreach via congressional leaders and President Biden *without* the support of other outside interlocuters marks an important pivot away from many community organizing models that either focus solely on tangential engagement with top-down stakeholders (e.g., voter drives, protests, awareness campaigns) or rely completely on outside funders (e.g., corporate funding, government lobbyist groups, professionalized activism). This liminal space is an undertheorized area for practitioners and researchers seeking to explore how communities build political agency while maintaining control of their own agendas and collective voice.

Another key insight encourages scholars and practitioners to reimagine definitions of what it means to be "radical" within grassroots campaigns. Historically, when people think of radical activist movement traditions, they are often accompanied by visions of disruption and direct action that seek to overturn the status quo and outright reject established institutions such as Marxism and the Labor Movement in Europe in the mid-to-late nineteenth century, the Black radical traditions during the 1960s Civil Rights era (e.g., Malcolm X, Black Panther Party), and the Stonewall Uprising in New York City in 1969. However, the narratives reflected in this book do not necessarily align with these traditions and upset conventional framings of how we understand radical organizing. For an outside observer, the women's "by any means necessary" approach to advocacy, which included working within existing legal, economic, and political structures, collaborating with conservative legislators, and using calculated idioms and language choices so as not to threaten dominant cultural hegemony might not seem radical on the surface. Yet, their positionalities as ACB women and core motivations for food justice were inherently radical and upset the status quo in that they subverted dominant narratives around who is allowed to shape policy and assert political agency. These strategies infuse nuanced perspectives for researchers and practitioners exploring the various dimensions of intersectional advocacy and political organizing in local and global contexts.

In a similar way, the book complicates romanticized portrayals of grassroots social justice projects as inherently autonomous, anti-establishment, and uniformly aligned in their philosophies and goals. Documenting the degree to which the women of NWIAA made calculated decisions around how to negotiate power, be seen as legitimate by external stakeholders, and simultaneously draw on shared cultural identities of marginalization on the one hand, but still not appear threatening to existing power structures on the other, brings to light the complex, microlevel realities of community activism that often get left out in romanticized and revisionist struggles for power. As evidenced across the women's narratives, their deep awareness of their marginalized social position allowed them to develop context-specific strategies that some may deem a comprise on the surface but were essential for them to meet their political goals. This builds on a growing body of political science research on Black communities' political engagement that underscores how they make rational and strategic decisions in voting behavior and policy advocacy (White & Laird, 2020; Wamble, 2025).

This is not to say that there is not tremendous potential for these types of grassroots-level organizing efforts as a catalyst to spur transformative food systems change—quite the opposite. The community represents an integral entry point for documenting what is happening on the ground in local contexts and across the world. Some of the most important social movements throughout history were born from ideas fostered in community-level mobilizing contexts. Beginning with and leveraging community voice to center cultural logics, lived realities, and localized knowledge and expertise will always be essential for intervention efforts to resonate with priority populations and bring multi-sector groups together. However, as documented in this text, without consistent monitoring and evaluating impact, these organizing efforts can become hamstrung by broader political barriers, interorganizational ambivalence, and underlying race, gender, and class tensions, complicating the potential of change efforts.

## The Road Ahead

The stories of the women featured in this book emerge alongside one of the most turbulent and politically divisive landscapes in recent memory. On November 6, 2024, former president Donald J. Trump won his re-election campaign for a second term in a surprisingly lopsided victory over then Vice President Kamala Harris, who was selected to run late after President Biden decided against a re-election bid. In the months leading up to the election, in what appeared to be a too-close-to-call, deadlocked race, Trump capitalized on an increasingly polarizing electorate to gain support by speaking to growing public perceptions around a declining national economy and progressive policies around immigration and social issues. Undergirded in much of Trump's rhetoric were strategic appeals to his political base, which ultimately served as consequential to the results of the election. The watershed moment presented an opportunity for the country to elect its first Black woman president, though most of American society quickly dismantled any likelihood of this possibility—justifying their decision by asserting that Harris was not qualified enough, did not have enough experience, and proposed too radical a political agenda. Relatedly, the women of NWIAA were all too familiar with how such cultural logics were used to establish a normative order that marked Black women as inferior and situated at the periphery.

The current political moment impacts all aspects of society and has the potential to influence decades of social progress. In the context of public health, the moment is particularly noteworthy given the arguments put forth in this book. At the time of this writing, President Trump appointed several cabinet positions to individuals who would help him strategically carry out his political and ideological visions. Arguably garnering the most attention is his appointment of Robert F. Kennedy, Jr., as Department of Health and Human Services secretary, which many experts argue could have important implications for public health policy and population health outcomes (Stolberg, 2025). While some of Kennedy Jr.'s immediate goals, such as cutting corporate influences out of FDA regulation, banning pesticides and GMO in agriculture, and limiting the use of food chemicals and additives in the national food supply, appear to align in principle and parrot the progressive agendas of many contemporary food justice and sovereignty movements—his implementation strategy, which includes an emphasis on rolling back federal regulatory processes and approach to practice which many in the science community have described as anti-science and evidence-based, has potential to drastically reshape existing public health systems and worsen health disparities, particularly among marginalized and under resourced communities. The public health workforce has largely panned the appointment and raised a flag for concern. For example, in the days immediately following the election results, the American Public Health Association released a public statement titled "Americans deserve better than RFK Jr" (APHA, 2024), where they opposed his appointment as Health and Human Services Secretary, citing his lack of medical and public health expertise, poor management qualifications, and history of spreading vaccine misinformation.

In the context of agriculture, President Trump appointed former White House aide Brooke Rollins to be the next Secretary of Agriculture on February 13, 2025. Rollins' previous role was President and CEO of the America First Policy Institute, a nonprofit think tank created in 2021 to promote Trump's public policy agenda. The Institute is the umbrella organization for America Legal First—the same public interest group largely responsible for overturning the 2021 Emergency Relief for Farmers of Color Act after alleging the federal government engaged in reverse discrimination. While in office, Rollins has promised to prioritize government deregulation and align the USDA with the principles of Trump's Department of Government Efficiency. Some of her early actions have included rescinding "all Diversity, Equity, Inclusion, and Accessibility (DEIA) programs to reprioritize unity, equality, and meritocracy" and the canceling of employee trainings, particularly those pertaining to "Environmental Justice and gender ideology" (USDA, 2025). These reforms are sure to have sweeping impacts for underrepresented farmer populations.

The Trump presidency has fostered several other national concerns, including a growing proximate connection with Project 2025, a sweeping political initiative published by the conservative think tank the Heritage Foundation. Central to the initiative is a focus on embedding conservative values into mainstream public health institutions such as the Centers for Disease Control and Prevention (CDC), National Institutes of Health (NIH), and the Food and Drug Administration (FDA), including the reevaluation of evidence-based practices, how funding gets allocated, and guiding health policies (Dans & Groves, 2023). These actions have already had impact during the administration's nascency, with wide-ranging executive actions such as imposing restrictions on the NIH,[1] banning all diversity, equity, and inclusion (DEI) programming in the federal workforce (including the USDA and FDA), cutting environmental justice programs at the Environmental Protection Agency and Department of Justice, among other mandates that have intersecting public health implications (Volcovici et al., 2025; Whitehouse.gov, 2025).

These actions have had wide-reaching global implications as well. For example, within his first month in office, President Trump issued an executive order freezing most US foreign aid for ninety days, in the process putting several humanitarian and development programs into a state of precarity (Joseph et al., 2025). More directly regarding public health and climate change, related executive actions including withdrawing the United States from the WHO and the Paris climate agreement have the potential to have indelible impacts on human and environmental health. If the breakneck pace of Trump's executive decision-making during his early moments in office is any indicator of

[1] Some of these restrictions have included implementing a hiring freeze, pausing official communications, banning travel, and slashing $4 billion from overheads in grants for biomedical research.

what his tenure will entail, the global future will undoubtedly remain in a perpetual state of uncertainty.

***

Despite this cavalcade of pressing challenges, ACB women remain on the front lines to advocate and support their local and global communities. For NWIAA, the political moment emerged at a pivotal time in their advocacy journey. After the primary data collection period for this project was completed, the organization experienced a mix of setbacks and triumphs in its quest to garner policy change. After several unsuccessful attempts to secure a meeting with President Biden to discuss their initial proposed charter bill, the women were forced to regroup and modify their existing political strategy. Still seeking to work within existing structures and garner external recognition by positioning themselves as "a subject of rights and a receiving body for state resources," NWIAA adapted their original "Equity and Inclusion" proposal to put more of an emphasis on women farmers specifically. After receiving co-sponsorship from Congresspeople Sheila Cherfilus-McCormick (D-FL), Congressman Jonathan L. Jackson (D-IL), Congresswoman Andrea Salinas (D-OR), and Congresswoman Julia Brownley (D-CA), their new bill—the Empowering Women in Agriculture Act (EWIAA; H.R. 9363)—was introduced to the US House of Representatives on August 16, 2024. The Act proposes "to amend the Food, Agriculture, Conservation, and Trade Act of 1990 to expand outreach and assistance to socially disadvantaged farmers and ranchers who are women, and for other purposes" (Congress.gov, 2024). Key goals of the EWIAA include allocating at least 10 percent of federal funds to women-focused organizations, including "women" in the definition of "socially disadvantaged farmers or ranchers" (Title 7 US Code § 2279), enhancing equitable access to resources for organizations serving disadvantaged farmers, and promoting gender equity by boosting opportunities for Black women and other underrepresented farmers (Cherfilus-McCormick, 2024). NWIAA hopes to get the bill passed under the Trump administration; at the time of this writing, the bill remains "introduced" to Congress with organizational leaders and various other advocates continuing to garner public and private support.

In many ways, this book ends where it began. The current political moment has relegated ACB women farmers to a familiar reality—the "1% of the 1%," far, few, in-between, and left to their own devices to secure resources and politically mobilize. However, the detailed political strategies, lived experiences, and shared knowledge of the women of NWIAA presented throughout the previous pages are not an exercise for naught. Rather, their innovative efforts to make transparent fractured ACB foodways and address food insecurity by connecting diasporic farming communities is an important contribution to scholarly inquiry and public health praxis. While this text only takes the reader as far as introducing NWIAA's model as a potential framework, it will be up to future practitioners and scholars to build upon these ideas and implement them in a more systematic and sustainable way.

# REFERENCES


Abah, D., & Naankiel, P. W. (2016). Structural adjustment programme in Nigeria and its implications on socio-economic development, 1980-1995. *The Calabar Historical Journal, 6*(2), 1–7.

Abubakar, I. B., Kankara, S. S., Malami, I., Danjuma, J. B., Muhammad, Y. Z., Yahaya, H., and Nurudeen, Q. O. (2022). Traditional medicinal plants used for treating emerging and re-emerging viral diseases in northern Nigeria. *European Journal of Integrative Medicine, 49*, 102094.

Adhikari, J. (2014). Seed sovereignty: Analysing the debate on hybrid seeds and GMOs and bringing about sustainability in agricultural development. *Journal of Forest and Livelihood, 12*(1), 33–46.

Agyemang, C., Bhopal, R., & Bruijnzeels, M. (2005). Negro, Black, Black African, African Caribbean, African American or what? Labelling African origin populations in the health arena in the 21st century. *Journal of Epidemiology & Community Health, 59*(12), 1014–1018.

Airhihenbuwa, C. O. (2007). *Healing our differences: The crisis of global health and the politics of identity*. Bloomsbury Publishing PLC.

Airhihenbuwa, C., & Dutta, M. (2012). New perspectives on global health communication. In R. Obregon & S. R. Waisbord (Eds.), *The handbook of global health communication* (pp. 34–51). Wiley-Blackwell.

Akamani, K. (2021). An ecosystem-based approach to climate-smart agriculture with some considerations for social equity. *Agronomy, 11*(8), 1564.

Al-Humaiqani, M. M., & Al-Ghamdi, S. G. (2023). Assessing the built environment's reflectivity, flexibility, resourcefulness, and rapidity resilience qualities against climate change impacts from the perspective of different stakeholders. *Sustainability*, 15(6), 5055.

Alkon, A., & Guthman, J. (Eds.). (2017). *The new food activism: Opposition, cooperation, and collective action*. University of California Press.

Alkon, A. H. (2012). *Black, white, and green: Farmers markets, race, and the green economy* (Vol. 13). University of Georgia Press.

Alkon, A. H., & Cadji, J. (2020). Sowing seeds of displacement: Gentrification and food justice in Oakland, CA. *International Journal of Urban and Regional Research, 44*(1), 108–123.

Alkon, A. H., & McCullen, C. G. (2011). Whiteness and farmers markets: Performances, perpetuations... contestations? *Antipode, 43*(4), 937–959.

Allen, P., & Guthman, J. (2006). From "old school" to "farm-to-school": Neoliberalization from the ground up. *Agriculture and Human Values, 23*, 401–415.

American Psychological Association (n.d.). Resilience. https://www.apa.org/topics/resilience

American Public Health Association (2024). *America deserves better than RFK Jr.* Retrieved from https://www.apha.org/news-and-media/news-releases/apha-news-releases/2024/rfk-jr-hhs-nomination

Anderson, M. D. (2021). How food in the commons can help to address inequity in US food and land access. *One Earth, 4*(2), 165–167.

Anderson, R. (2016). Afrofuturism 2.0 & the Black speculative arts movement: Notes on a manifesto. *Obsidian, 42*(1/2), 228–236.

Andrulis, D. P. (1998). Access to care is the centerpiece in the elimination of socioeconomic disparities in health. *Annals of Internal Medicine, 129*(5), 412–416.

Austin, G. (2009). Cash crops and freedom: Export agriculture and the decline of slavery in colonial West Africa. *International Review of Social History, 54*(1), 1–37.

Baba, I. B., Zain, R. M., Idris, H. U., & Sanni, A. N. (2015). The role of women in household decision-making and their contribution to agriculture and rural development in Nigeria. *IOSR Journal of Humanities and Social Science, 20*(5), 30–39.

Babb, A., Betz, M., Pahk, S. H., & Smith, I. (2023). Nostalgia and the protection of white supremacy at a public farmers' market. *Gastronomica: The Journal of Food and Culture, 23*(2), 84–94.

Bagdonis, J. M., Hinrichs, C. C., & Schafft, K. A. (2009). The emergence and framing of farm-to-school initiatives: Civic engagement, health and local agriculture. *Agriculture and Human Values, 26*, 107–119.

Bailey, C., & Thomson, R. (2022). Heirs property, critical race theory, and reparations. *Rural Sociology, 87*(4), 1219–1243.

Barry, T., & Gahman, L. (2020). Agrarian struggle and food system injustice in the Anglo-Caribbean: Centering social reproduction by (re) turning to Creft and Fanon. *Human Geography, 13*(2), 174–178.

Barry, T., & Gahman, L. (2021). Food system and social reproduction realities for women in agriculture across the Caribbean: Evidence from Grenada, St. Lucia, and St. Vincent and the Grenadines. *Journal of Agrarian Change, 21*(4), 815–833.

Barry, T., Gahman, L., Greenidge, A., & Mohamed, A. (2020). Wrestling with race and colonialism in Caribbean agriculture: Toward a (food) sovereign and (gender) just future. *Geoforum, 109*, 106–110.

Beinart, W. (2000). African history and environmental history. *African Affairs, 99*(395), 269–302.

Beinart, W., & Hughes, L. (2007). *Environment and empire.* Oxford University Press.

Benjamin, R. (2020). *Black skin, white masks: Racism, vulnerability, & refuting Black pathology.* Department of African American Studies, Princeton University.

Bikomeye, J. C., Namin, S., Anyanwu, C., Rublee, C. S., Ferschinger, J., Leinbach, K., and Beyer, K. M. (2021). Resilience and equity in a time of crises: Investing in public urban greenspace is now more essential than ever in the US and beyond. *International Journal of Environmental Research and Public Health, 18*(16), 8420.

Bill & Melinda Gates Foundation (2024). *Agricultural development.* https://www.gatesfoundation.org/our-work/programs/global-growth-and-opportunity/agricultural-development

Binder, C., & Binder, C. (2016). A capability perspective on indigenous autonomy. *Oxford Development Studies, 44*(3), 297–314.

Black, T. (2016). Race, gender, and climate injustice: dimensions of social and environmental inequality. In P. Godfrey & D. Torres (Eds.), *Systemic Crises of Global Climate Change* (pp. 172–184). Routledge.

Blaut, J. M., Mark, F. X., & Dammann, A. E. (1965). *Report to the governor of the United States Virgin Islands on the reconstruction of the agriculture economy of St. Croix, Virgin Islands.* College of the Virgin Islands, Caribbean Research Institute.

Bolin, A. (2024). "They don't care about Crucian culture": Legitimising claims to heritage rights in St. Croix, US Virgin Islands. *International Journal of Heritage Studies, 30*(7), 784–798.

Bonds, A. (2018). Refusing resilience: The racialization of risk and resilience. *Urban Geography, 39*(8), 1285–1291.

Borg, S. (2024). "A battle for the soul of this nation": How domestic polarization affects US foreign policy in post-Trump America. *International Journal, 79*(1), 22–39.

Borras, A. M., & Mohamed, F. A. (2020). Health inequities and the shifting paradigms of food security, food insecurity, and food sovereignty. *International Journal of Health Services, 50*(3), 299–313.

Bowdler, J. A. (2021). *The countercultural back-to-the-land movement.* University of Washington.

Bowens, N. (2015). *The color of food: Stories of race, resilience and farming.* New Society Publisher.

Breilh, J. (2021). *Critical epidemiology and the people's health.* Oxford University Press.

Brixiová, Z., Kangoye, T., & Tregenna, F. (2020). Enterprising women in Southern Africa: When does land ownership matter? *Journal of Family and Economic Issues, 41*(1), 37–51.

Broad, G. (2016). *More than just food: Food justice and community change* (Vol. 60). University of California Press.

Brown, N. E. (2014). *Sisters in the statehouse: Black women and legislative decision making.* Oxford University Press.

Bustillo, X. (2023). In 2022, Black farmers were persistently left behind from the USDA's loan system. *NPR KQED.* https://www.npr.org/2023/02/19/1156851675/in-2022-black-farmers-were-persistently-left-behind-from-the-usdas-loan-system

Cachelin, A., Ivkovich, L., Jensen, P., & Neild, M. (2019). Leveraging foodways for health and justice. *Local Environment, 24*(5), 417–427.

Canfield, M. (2022). The ideology of innovation: Philanthropy and racial capitalism in global food governance. *The Journal of Peasant Studies, 50*(6), 2381–2405.

Cannuscio, C. C., Weiss, E. E., & Asch, D. A. (2010). The contribution of urban foodways to health disparities. *Journal of Urban Health, 87*, 381–393.

Carcamo, P., Brugler, S., & Sahraei, M. (2023). *Artificial Intelligence applications in agriculture need a justice lens to address risks and provide benefits to smallholder farmers.* United Nations' Sustainable Development Goals Knowledge Platform.

Carney, J. A. (2001). African rice in the Columbian Exchange. *Journal of African History, 42*(3), 377–396.

Carney, J. A. (2009). *Black rice: The African origins of rice cultivation in the Americas.* Harvard University Press.

Carroll, F. (2014). The racial politics of place: Jim Crow, the New Deal, and suburban housing on the Virginia Peninsula. *Journal of Urban History, 40*(3), 514–535.

Carter, A., Broad, G., & Reeves, V. (2024). Recapturing communicative erasure: Black women farmers' lived experience, political voice and cultural knowledge as critical health communication praxis. *Health Communication, 40*(1), 3–14.

Carter, A. L., & Alexander, A. (2020). Soul food: [Re] framing the African-American farming crisis using the culture-centered approach. *Frontiers in Communication, 5*, 5.

Carter-Edwards, L., Hooten, E. G., Bruce, M. A., Toms, F., Lloyd, C. L., & Ellison, C. (2012). Pilgrimage to wellness: An exploratory report of rural African American clergy perceptions of church health promotion capacity. *Journal of Prevention & Intervention in the Community, 40*(3), 194–207.

Chae, D. H., Snipes, S. A., Chung, K. W., Martz, C. D., & LaVeist, T. A. (2021). Vulnerability and resilience: Use and misuse of these terms in the public health discourse. *American Journal of Public Health, 111*(10), 1736–1740.

Chandanabhumma, P. P., Duran, B. M., Peterson, J. C., Pearson, C. R., Oetzel, J. G., Dutta, M. J., & Wallerstein, N. B. (2019). Space within the scientific discourse for the voice of the other? Expressions of community voice in the scientific discourse of community-based participatory research. *Health Communication, 35*(5), 616–627.

Chang, D. A. (2010). *The color of the land: Race, nation, and the politics of landownership in Oklahoma, 1832-1929*. University of North Carolina Press.

Chávez, V., Duran, B., Baker, Q. E., Avila, M. M., & Wallerstein, N. (2008). The dance of race and privilege in CBPR. In M. Minkler & N. Wallerstein (Eds.), *Community-based participatory research for health: From process to outcomes* (pp. 91–105).

Cherfilus-McCormick, S. (2024). Reps. Cherfilus-McCormick, Jackson, Brownley, and Salinas introduce the "Empowering Women in Agriculture Act." https://cherfilus-mccormick.house.gov/media/press-releases/reps-cherfilus-mccormick-jackson-brownley-and-salinas-introduce-empowering

Clifford, A., Lang, L., Chen, R., Anstey, K. J., & Seaton, A. (2016). Exposure to air pollution and cognitive functioning across the life course–a systematic literature review. *Environmental Research, 147*, 383–398.

Coaffee, J., & Rogers, P. (2008). Rebordering the city for new security challenges: From counter-terrorism to community resilience. *Space and Polity, 12*(1), 101–118.

Cohen, C. J. (2009). *The boundaries of blackness: AIDS and the breakdown of black politics*. University of Chicago Press.

Coleman-Jensen, A., Rabbitt, M. P., Gregory, C. A., & Singh, A. (2021). Household food security in the United States in 2020. USDA Economic Revenue Service. https://www.ers.usda.gov/publications/pub-details?pubid=104655&utm

Coleman-Jensen, G., Rabbitt, M., Gregory, C. & Singh, A. (2016). Household food security in the United States in 2015. USDA Economic Revenue Service. https://www.ers.usda.gov/publications/pub-details?pubid=79760

Colson-Fearon, B., & Versey, H. S. (2022). Urban agriculture as a means to food sovereignty? A case study of Baltimore city residents. *International Journal of Environmental Research and Public Health, 19*(19), 12752.

Congress.gov (2021). H.R.40 - commission to study and develop reparation proposals for African Americans Act. https://www.congress.gov/bill/117th-congress/house-bill/40

Congress.gov (2023). Justice for Black farmers act, H.R. 1167, 118th Congress. https://www.congress.gov/118/bills/hr1167/BILLS-118hr1167ih.pdf

Congress.gov (2024). H.R.9363 - Empowering Women in Agriculture Act. https://www.congress.gov/bill/118th-congress/house-bill/9363/text/ih

Congressional Research Service (2023). USDA nutrition assistance programs: Response to the COVID-19 pandemic. https://crsreports.congress.gov/product/pdf/R/R46681

Conquergood, D. (2002). Performance studies: Interventions and radical research. *TDR/The Drama Review, 46*(2), 145–156.

Conrad, A., & Zuckerman, J. (2020). *Identifying and countering White supremacy culture in food systems.* Duke Sanford World Food Policy Center.

Cooley, A. J. (2015). *To live and dine in Dixie: The evolution of urban food culture in the Jim Crow South* (Vol. 8). University of Georgia Press.

Copeland, R. W. (1984). The rise and fall of Black real property ownership: A review of Black land ownership from the rough beginnings to the great gains; dispossession via the use of legal tactics and the push for Black land retention. *Black LJ, 9*, 51.

Copeland, R. W. (2015). Heir property in the African American community: From promised lands to problem lands. *Professional Agricultural Workers Journal, 2*(2), 2.

Creswell, J. W. (1998). *Qualitative inquiry and research design: Choosing among five traditions.* Sage Publications.

Crisp, B. F., & Kelly, M. J. (1999). The socioeconomic impacts of structural adjustment. *International Studies Quarterly, 43*(3), 533–552.

Crossman, S., Robles, C., Stanley, D., & Petersen, L. (2010). The "Virgin Fresh" apicultural project: Development and expansion of the U.S. Virgin Islands apiculture industry. In *Paper presented at the 46th Annual Meeting of the Caribbean Food Crops Society, Boca Chica, Dominican Republic.* Caribbean Food Crops Society.

D'Odorico, P., Carr, J. A., Davis, K. F., Dell'Angelo, J., & Seekell, D. A. (2019). Food inequality, injustice, and rights. *BioScience, 69*(3), 180–190.

Dabone, C., Mbagwu, I., Muray, M., Ubangha, L., Kohoun, B., Etowa, E, and Etowa, J. (2021). Global food insecurity and African, Caribbean, and Black (ACB) populations during the COVID-19 pandemic: A rapid review. *Journal of Racial and Ethnic Health Disparities, 9*(2), 420–435.

Dachaga, W., & de Vries, W. T. (2022). Integrating urban land tenure security in health determinants: The design of indicators for measuring land tenure security and health relationships in developing country contexts. *International Journal of Environmental Research and Public Health, 19*(5), 3080.

Daniel, P. (2013). *Dispossession: Discrimination against African American farmers in the age of civil rights.* UNC Press Books.

Daniel, P. (1985). *Breaking the land: The transformation of cotton, tobacco, and rice cultures since 1880*. University of Illinois Press.

Dans, P., & Groves, S. (Eds.). (2023). *Mandate for leadership: The conversative promise*. The Heritage Foundation.

Darity Jr., W. (2008). Forty acres and a mule in the 21st century. *Social Science Quarterly, 89*(3), 656–664.

Darity, W., Jr., & Nicholson, M. J. (2005). Racial wealth inequality and the Black family. In V. C. McLoyd, N. E. Hill & K. A. Dodge (Eds.), *African American family life: Ecological and cultural diversity* (pp. 78–85). The Guilford Press.

Darnhofer, I., Lamine, C., Strauss, A., & Navarrete, M. (2016). The resilience of family farms: Towards a relational approach. *Journal of Rural Studies, 44*, 111–122.

Davidson, J. L., Jacobson, C., Lyth, A., Dedekorkut-Howes, A., Baldwin, C. L., Ellison, J. C., and Smith, T. F. (2016). Interrogating resilience: Toward a typology to improve its operationalization. *Ecology and Society, 21*(2), 27.

De Souza, R. T. (2019). *Feeding the other: Whiteness, privilege, and neoliberal stigma in food pantries*. MIT Press.

De Souza, R. (2024). Women in the margins: A culture-centered interrogation of hunger and "food apartheid" in the United States. *Health Communication, 39*(9), 1855–1865.

Deb, S. (2020). W.N.B.A. players escalate protest of anti-B.L.M. team owner. *The New York Times*. https://www.nytimes.com/2020/08/04/sports/basketball/wnba-dream-loeffler-warnock.html

Depew, B., Fishback, P. V., & Rhode, P. W. (2013). New deal or no deal in the Cotton South: The effect of the AAA on the agricultural labor structure. *Explorations in Economic History, 50*(4), 466–486.

Derickson, K. D. (2016). Resilience is not enough. *City, 20*(1), 161–166.

Devine, C. M. (2005). A life course perspective: Understanding food choices in time, social location, and history. *Journal of Nutrition Education and Behavior, 37*(3), 121–128.

De Zwart, P., & Van Zanden, J. L. (2018). *The origins of globalization: World trade in the making of the global economy, 1500-1800*. Cambridge University Press.

Dray, P. (2007). *At the hands of persons unknown: The lynching of Black America*. Modern Library.

Dutta, M. (2020). *Communication, culture and social change: Meaning, co-option and resistance*. Springer International Publishing.

Dutta, M. J. (2018). Culture-centered approach in addressing health disparities: Communication infrastructures for subaltern voices. *Communication Methods and Measures, 12*(4), 239–259.

Dutta, M. J. (2024). Decolonizing the pedagogy of health communication campaigns: A culture-centered approach. *Communication Education, 73*(4), 405–426.

Dutta, M. J., & Basu, A. (2011). Culture, communication, and health: A guiding framework. In T. L. Thompson, R. Parrott & J. F. Nussbaum (Eds.), *The Routledge handbook of health communication* (pp. 346–360). Routledge.

Dutta, M. J., Mandal, I., Kaur, S., Pitaloka, D., Pandi, A., Tan, N., ..., & Sastry, S. (2016). *Culture-centered method: The nuts and bolts of co-creating communication infrastructures of listening in communities.* The Center for Culture-Centered Approach to Research and Evaluation (CARE), National University of Singapore.

Dyer, J. F., Bailey, C., & Tran, N. V. (2008). Ownership characteristics of heir property in a Black Belt county: A quantitative approach. *Journal of Rural Social Sciences, 24*(2), 10.

Ebbinghaus, M., Bailey, N., & Rubel, J. (2024). The effect of the 2020 Black lives matter protests on police budgets: How "Defund the Police" sparked political backlash. *Social Problems, 72*(3), 1198–1215.

Edmonstone, W. (2024). The modern plantation empire and Eric Walrond's tropic death. *Twentieth Century Literature, 70*(2), 95–126.

Egid, B. R., Roura, M., Aktar, B., Quach, J. A., Chumo, I., Dias, S., and Ozano, K. (2021). "You want to deal with power while riding on power": Global perspectives on power in participatory health research and co-production approaches. *BMJ Global Health, 6*(11), e006978.

Ellis, W. R., & Dietz, W. H. (2017). A new framework for addressing adverse childhood and community experiences: The building community resilience model. *Academic Pediatrics, 17*(7), S86–S93.

Escobar, A. (2008) *Territories of difference: Place, movements, life, redes.* Duke University Press.

Evans, J. P. (2011). Resilience, ecology and adaptation in the experimental city. *Transactions of the institute of British Geographers, 36*(2), 223–237.

Everbach, T., Nisbett, G. S., & Weiller-Abels, K. (2022). The WNBA and Black women athletes' social activism. In A. M. Colombo-Dougovito, T. Everbach & K. Weiller-Abels (Eds.), *Not playing around: Intersectional identities, media representation, and the power of sport* (pp. 143–161). Lexington Books.

Farmer, A. D. (2017). *Remaking Black power: How Black women transformed an era.* UNC Press Books.

Fields-Black, E. L. (2008). *Deep roots: Rice farmers in West Africa and the African diaspora.* Indiana University Press.

Folsom, B. W., Jr. (2009). *New Deal or raw deal?: How FDR's economic legacy has damaged America.* Simon and Schuster.

Foner, E. (1988). Reconstruction: America's unfinished revolution, 1863-1877. In *New American nation series* (Vol. 51, p. 29). Harper & Row Publishers.

Food and Agriculture Organization of the United Nations. (2011). *Global food losses and food waste – Extent, causes and prevention.* Rome, FAO.

Food and Agriculture Organization of the United Nations. (2022). *The state of food security and nutrition in the world 2022. Repurposing food and agricultural policies to make healthy diets more affordable.* Rome, FAO.

Forson, P. W., & Counihan, C. (2013). *Taking food public: Redefining foodways in a changing world.* Routledge.

Fortenberry, B. R. (2021). Heritage justice, conservation, and tourism in the greater Caribbean. In T. Jamal & J. Higham (Eds.), *Justice and tourism: Principles and approaches for local-global sustainability and well-being* (pp. 111–134). Routledge.

Francis, D. V., Hamilton, D., Mitchell, T. W., Rosenberg, N. A., & Stucki, B. W. (2022). Black land loss: 1920–1997. *AEA Papers and Proceedings, 112*, 38–42.

Fraser, N. (1996). *Justice interruptus: Critical reflections on the "postsocialist" condition.* Routledge.

Fry, W., Koseff, A., & Kamal, S. (2024). Two historic California reparations bills stall out— sparing Newsom a tough political call. *Cal Matters.* https://calmatters.org/california-divide/2024/08/california-reparations-bills-3/

Galaz, V., Centeno, M. A., Callahan, P. W., Causevic, A., Patterson, T., Brass, I., ... & Levy, K. (2021). Artificial intelligence, systemic risks, and sustainability. *Technology in Society, 67*, 101741.

Galli, S., Theodoridis, D., & Rönnbäck, K. (2024). Elite persistence and inequality in the Danish West Indies, 1760–1914. *Explorations in Economic History, 94*, 101636.

Ganti, T. (2014). Neoliberalism. *Annual Review of Anthropology, 43*(1), 89–104.

Georgia General Assembly (2024). HR 1341 Whitehead, Noreen S.; commend. https://www.legis.ga.gov/legislation/68641

Gilbert, J., Sharp, G., & Felin, M. S. (2002). The loss and persistence of black-owned farms and farmland: A review of the research literature and its implications. *Journal of Rural Social Sciences, 18*(2), 1.

Gordon, C., Hunt, K. P., & Dutta, M. J. (2022). Food systems communication amid compounding crises: Power, resistance, and change. *Frontiers in Communication, 7*, 1041474.

Granovetter, M. S. (1973). The strength of weak ties. *American Journal of Sociology, 78*(6), 1360–1380.

Grant, G. R., Wood, S. D., & Wright, W. J. (2012). Black farmers united: The struggle against power and principalities. *Journal of Pan African Studies, 5*(1), 3–22.

Green, C. A. (2006). Between respectability and self-respect: Framing Afro-Caribbean women's labour history. *Social and Economic Studies, 55*(3), 1–31.

Grefe, E. A. (1997). Grassroots or grasstops: Your call . . . your gamble. *Economic Development Review, 15*(2), 15.

Griffin, R. A., & Rossing, J. P. (2020). Black Panther in widescreen: cross-disciplinary perspectives on a pioneering, paradoxical film. *Review of Communication, 20*(3), 203–219.

Grove, K., Cox, S., & Barnett, A. (2020). Racializing resilience: Assemblage, critique, and contested futures in greater Miami resilience planning. *Annals of the American Association of Geographers, 110*(5), 1613–1630.

Gruver, J., Lee, K., & Hayes, E. (2024). Food insecurity in paradise: An exploration of food system resilience in the US Virgin Islands. *Journal of Agriculture, Food Systems, and Community Development, 14*(1), 1–19.

Guannel, G., Lohmann, H., & Dwyer, J. (2022). *The public health implications of social vulnerability in the U.S. Virgin Islands.* Natural Hazards Center. https://hazards.colorado.edu/public-health-disaster-research/the-public-health-implications-of-social-vulnerability-in-the-u-s-virgin-islands

Gugliotta, G. (1990). Dwindling Black farmers fight formidable odds for future: Agriculture: Small operations, particularly those owned by African-Americans, are disappearing. Their numbers have declined from one-seventh in 1920 to less than 1% today. *Los Angeles Times.* https://www.latimes.com/archives/la-xpm-1990-12-30-mn-10124-story.html

Guthman, J. (2003). Fast food/organic food: Reflexive tastes and the making of "yuppie chow". *Social & Cultural Geography, 4*(1), 45–58.

Guthman, J. (2011). If they only knew: The unbearable whiteness of alternative food. In A. H. Alkon & J. Agyeman (Eds.), *Cultivating food justice: race, class and sustainability* (pp. 263–281). The MIT Press.

Hague, J. (April 26, 2023). Women's basketball is raking in more cash than ever, but the players aren't: WNBA base salaries as a share of revenue have shrunk, despite the league's rapid growth. *Bloomberg.* https://www.bloomberg.com/news/features/2023-04-26/wnba-is-growing-but-players-aren-t-getting-a-penny-of-revenue-share?embedded-checkout=true

Halcrow, E. M. (1982). *Canes and chains: A study of sugar and slavery* (Vol. 3). Heinemann.

Hall, C. (2020). Editorial: Black women got Biden elected. Of course they did. *Los Angeles Times.* https://www.latimes.com/opinion/story/2020-11-25/editorial-black-women-got-biden-elected-of-course-they-did

Harper, A. B. (Ed.). (2009). *Sistah vegan: Black female vegans speak on food, identity, health, and society.* Lantern Books.

Harper, A. B. (2011). The absence of meat in Oankali dietary philosophy: An eco-feminist-vegan analysis of Octavia Butler's Dawn. In S. Jackson & J. E. Moody-Freeman (Eds.), *The Black imagination: Science fiction, futurism and the speculative* (pp. 111–129). Routledge.

Harrigan, N., & Varlack, P. I. (1977). The US Virgin Islands and the black experience. *Journal of Black Studies, 7*(4), 387–410.

Harris, C. V. (2009). "Well I just generally bes the president of everything": Rural Black women's empowerment through South Carolina home demonstration activities. *Black Women, Gender & Families, 3*(1), 91–112.

Hassel, C. A. (2014). Reconsidering nutrition science: Critical reflection with a cultural lens. *Nutrition Journal, 13*, 1–11.

Hausman, J. K., Rhode, P. W., & Wieland, J. F. (2021). Farm product prices, redistribution, and the early US Great depression. *The Journal of Economic History, 81*(3), 649–687.

Hayes, J. (2021). Timeline: Black farmers and the USDA. In *Environmental working group*. https://www.ewg.org/research/timeline-black-farmers-and-usda

Hayes, M., & Hibbing, M. V. (2017). The symbolic benefits of descriptive and substantive representation. *Political Behavior, 39*, 31–50.

Hayes-Conroy, A. (Ed.). (2016). *Doing nutrition differently: Critical approaches to diet and dietary intervention*. Routledge.

Hedberg, R. C. (2021). An instrumental-reflexive approach to assessing and building food system resilience. *Geography Compass, 15*(7), e12581.

Heidhues, F., & Obare, G. A. (2011). Lessons from structural adjustment programmes and their effects in Africa. *Quarterly Journal of International Agriculture, 50*(1), 55–64.

Helfrich, J. T., Oberg, M. L., Roberts, A. E., Reed, J. L., & Bruyneel, K. (2021). No more nations within nations: Indigenous sovereignty after the end of treaty-making in 1871. *The Journal of the Gilded Age and Progressive Era, 20*(2), 325–329.

Herlitz, L., MacIntyre, H., Osborn, T., & Bonell, C. (2020). The sustainability of public health interventions in schools: A systematic review. *Implementation Science, 15*, 1–28.

Herman, D. R., Taylor Baer, M., Adams, E., Cunningham-Sabo, L., Duran, N., Johnson, D. B., & Yakes, E. (2014). Life course perspective: Evidence for the role of nutrition. *Maternal and Child Health Journal, 18*, 450–461.

Hilal, S., & Brayne, C. (2022). Epidemiologic trends, social determinants, and brain health: The role of life course inequalities. *Stroke, 53*(2), 437–443.

Hill-Collins, P. (2000). *Black feminist thought: Knowledge, consciousness, and the politics of empowerment*. Routledge.

Hing, A. K., Chantarat, T., Fashaw-Walters, S., Hunt, S. L., & Hardeman, R. R. (2024). Instruments for racial health equity: A scoping review of structural racism measurement, 2019-2021. *Epidemiologic Reviews, 46*(1), 1–26.

Hinson, W. R., & Robinson, E. (2008). "We didn't get nothing:" The plight of Black farmers. *Journal of African American Studies, 12*, 283–302.

Hite, A. H., & Carter, A. (2019). Examining assumptions in science-based policy: Critical health communication, stasis theory, and public health nutrition guidance. *Rhetoric of Health & Medicine*, *2*(2), 147–175.

Ho, E. Y., & Sharf, B. F. (2021). Cultural theories of health communication. In T. L. Thompson & P. J. Schulz (Eds.), *Health communication theory* (pp. 278–299). Wiley.

Holden, L. (2024). California slavery reparations bills unraveled over Gavin Newsom amendments. *Politico*. https://www.politico.com/news/2024/08/31/california-slavery-reparations-bills-unraveled-over-gavin-newsom-amendments-00176957

Holmes, A. G. D. (2020). Researcher positionality—A consideration of its influence and place in qualitative research—A new researcher guide. *Shanlax International Journal of Education*, *8*(4), 1–10.

Holt Giménez, E., & Shattuck, A. (2011). Food crises, food regimes and food movements: rumblings of reform or tides of transformation? *The Journal of Peasant Studies*, *38*(1), 109–144.

Hooks, B. (1997). Sisterhood: Political solidarity between women. In D. T. Meyers (Ed.), *Feminist social thought: A reader* (pp. 484–501). Routledge.

Hoppe, T. A., Litovitz, A., Willis, K. A., Meseroll, R. A., Perkins, M. J., Hutchins, B. I., ... & Santangelo, G. M. (2019). Topic choice contributes to the lower rate of NIH awards to African-American/Black scientists. *Science Advances*, *5*(10), eaaw7238.

Horst, M., & Marion, A. (2019). Racial, ethnic and gender inequities in farmland ownership and farming in the US. *Agriculture and Human Values*, *36*, 1–16.

Housel, J., Saxen, C., & Wahlrab, T. (2018). Experiencing intentional recognition: Welcoming immigrants in Dayton, Ohio. *Urban Studies*, *55*(2), 384–405.

Hubbard, K. K. (2019). The sobering details behind the latest seed monopoly chart. *Civil Eats*. https://civileats.com/2019/01/11/the-sobering-details-behind-the-latest-seed-monopoly-chart/

Hume, C., Grieger, J. A., Kalamkarian, A., D'Onise, K., & Smithers, L. G. (2022). Community gardens and their effects on diet, health, psychosocial and community outcomes: A systematic review. *BMC Public Health*, *22*(1), 1247.

Hutcheon, E., & Lashewicz, B. (2014). Theorizing resilience: Critiquing and unbounding a marginalizing concept. *Disability & Society*, *29*(9), 1383–1397.

Iwelunmor, J., Newsome, V., & Airhihenbuwa, C. O. (2014). Framing the impact of culture on health: A systematic review of the PEN-3 cultural model and its application in public health research and interventions. *Ethnicity & Health*, *19*(1), 20–46.

Jalata, A. (2013). Colonial terrorism, global capitalism and African underdevelopment: 500 years of crimes against African peoples. *The Journal of Pan African Studies*, *5*(9), 1–42.

James, D. (2020). *Philanthropy and race in the US Virgin Islands*. St. Croix Foundation for Community Development.

Jan, T., McGregor, J., & Hoyer, M. (2021). Corporate America's $50 billion promise: A post analysis of racial justice pledges after George Floyd's death reveals the limits of corporate power to effect change. *The Washington Post*. https://www.washingtonpost.com/business/interactive/2021/george-floyd-corporate-america-racial-justice/

Johnson, C., Dowd, T. J., & Ridgeway, C. L. (2006). Legitimacy as a social process. *Annual Review of Sociology 32*(1), 53–78.

Jones, L. (2019). Resilience isn't the same for all: Comparing subjective and objective approaches to resilience measurement. *Wiley Interdisciplinary Reviews: Climate Change*, *10*(1), e552.

Jones, M. S. (2020). *Vanguard: How Black women broke barriers, won the vote, and insisted on equality for all*. Basic Books.

Jordan, W. D. (2013). *White over black: American attitudes toward the Negro, 1550-1812*. UNC Press Books.

Joseph, Y., Khurana, M., & Pasick, A. (2025). Trump's foreign aid freeze has created chaos. Here is what to know. *New York Times*. https://www.nytimes.com/article/us-foreign-aid-freeze-explained.html

Kanu, I. A., & Ndubisi, E. (Eds.). (2020). *African Indigenous knowledge systems: Problems and perspectives*. Association for the Promotion of African Studies.

Kawachi, A. R. (2022). Municipal fair housing act litigation and reparations. *UCLA Law Review*, *69*, 1322.

Kim, H. S., Kim H. J., & Juon, H. S. (2021). Racial/ethnic disparities in patient-provider communication and the role of e-health use. *Journal of Health Communication*, *26*(3), 194–203.

Kimura, A. H., Biltekoff, C., Mudry, J., & Hayes-Conroy, J. (2014). Nutrition as a project. *Gastronomica: The Journal of Food and Culture*, *14*(3), 34–45.

Kolavalli, C. (2020). Confronting whiteness in Kansas City's local food movement: Diversity work and discourse on privilege and power. *Gastronomica*, *20*(1), 59–68.

Kondo, C., Zollet, S., Kobayashi, M., & Yamamoto, N. (2024). Fifty years of Teikei: The evolution of the movement's ten principles and its impact on alternative food initiatives in Japan. *Frontiers in Sustainable Food Systems*, *8*, 1368253.

Kutlaca, M., & Radke, H. R. (2023). Towards an understanding of performative allyship: Definition, antecedents and consequences. *Social and Personality Psychology Compass*, *17*(2), e12724.

Laborde, D., Martin, W., Swinnen, J., & Vos, R. (2020). COVID-19 risks to global food security. *Science*, *369*(6503), 500–502.

Lanza, M. L. (1999). *Agrarianism and reconstruction politics: The Southern Homestead Act*. LSU Press.

Larimore, S. (2018). Cultural boundaries to access in farmers markets accepting Supplemental Nutrition Assistance Program (SNAP). *Qualitative Sociology*, *41*(1), 63–87.

Layman, E., & Civita, N. (2022). Decolonizing agriculture in the United States: Centering the knowledges of women and people of color to support relational farming practices. *Agriculture and Human Values*, *39*(3), 965–978.

Leach, M., Rockström, J., Raskin, P., Scoones, I., Stirling, A. C., Smith, A., ... & Olsson, P. (2012). Transforming innovation for sustainability. *Ecology and Society*, *17*(2), 11.

Lee, L. H., & Abdullah, Z. (2024). Antecedents of internal reputation and its consequences on organizational outcomes: A systematic review. *International Journal of Organization Theory & Behavior*, *27*(1), 55–79.

Leeds-Hurwitz, W. (2016). Urban foodways as communication and intangible cultural heritage. In *Urban foodways and communication: Ethnographic studies in intangible culture food heritages around the world* (pp. 185–200). Bloomsbury Publishing.

Leslie, I. S., Wypler, J., & Bell, M. M. (2019). Relational agriculture: Gender, sexuality, and sustainability in US farming. *Society & Natural Resources*, *32*(8), 853–874.

Lett, E., Adekunle, D., McMurray, P., Asabor, E. N., Irie, W., Simon, M. A., ... & McLemore, M. R. (2022). Health equity tourism: Ravaging the justice landscape. *Journal of Medical Systems*, *46*(3), 17.

Levenson, M. (2021). Judge blocks $4 billion U.S. debt relief program for minority farmers. *The New York Times*. https://www.nytimes.com/2021/06/23/us/politics/biden-debt-relief-black-farmers.html

Levkoe, C. Z., & Offeh-Gyimah, A. (2020). Race, privilege and the exclusivity of farm internships: Ecological agricultural education and the implications for food movements. *Environment and Planning E: Nature and Space*, *3*(2), 580–598.

Lewis, J. S., Bradford, S., Holder, L., Montgomery Steppe, M., Grills, C., Tamaki, D. K., ... Moore, K. V. (2023). *The California reparations report*. The State of California.

Lim, J. J., Kim, Y. C., & Koch-Weser, S. (2022). Catalyzing storytelling in communication infrastructure theory: A study of local ethnic media. *Journal of Health Communication*, *27*(5), 312–325.

Lindemann, J., Alter, T. R., Stagner, F., Palacios, E., Banuna, L., & Muldoon, M. (2022). Building urban community resilience through university extension:

Community engagement and the politics of knowledge. *Socio-Ecological Practice Research, 4*(4), 325–337.

Littlefield, D. C. (1991). *Rice and slaves: Ethnicity and the slave trade in colonial South Carolina.* University of Illinois Press.

Litwack, L. F. (2009). *How free is free?: The long death of Jim Crow* (Vol. 6). Harvard University Press.

Lohnes, J., & Pine, A. (2023). Feeding lines: Standing up in the neoliberal charitable food regime. *Human Geography, 16*(2), 212–220.

Lowery, W. (2023). *American whitelash.* Harper Collins.

Lu, A. J., Sannon, S., Moy, C., Brewer, S., Green, J., Jackson, K. N., ... & Dillahunt, T. R. (2023). Shifting from surveillance-as-safety to safety-through-noticing: A photovoice study with Eastside Detroit residents. In *Proceedings of the 2023 CHI Conference on Human Factors in Computing Systems* (pp. 1–19).

Lunsford, L., Arthur, M. L., & Porter, C. M. (2021). African and Native American foodways and resilience: From 1619 to COVID-19. *Journal of Agriculture, Food Systems, and Community Development, 10*(4), 241.

Mackenzie, J., & Murray, E. (2021). Socially constructing healthy eating: A Foucauldian discourse analysis of healthy eating information and advice. *Qualitative Health Research, 31*(11), 2135–2146.

MacKinnon, D., & Derickson, K. D. (2013). From resilience to resourcefulness: A critique of resilience policy and activism. *Progress in Human Geography, 37*(2), 253–270.

Madison, D. S. (2011). *Critical ethnography: Method, ethics, and performance.* Sage publications.

Mapara, J. (2009). Indigenous knowledge systems in Zimbabwe: Juxtaposing postcolonial theory. *Journal of Pan African Studies, 3*(1), 139–155.

Marfurt, F., Haller, T., & Bottazzi, P. (2023). Green agendas and white markets: The coloniality of agroecology in Senegal. *Land, 12*(7), 1324.

Marrero, A., & Mattei, J. (2022). Reclaiming traditional, plant-based, climate-resilient food systems in small islands. *The Lancet Planetary Health, 6*(2), e171–e179.

Marsh, C. E. (1981). A socio-historical analysis of the Labor Revolt of 1878 in the Danish West Indies. *Phylon (1960-), 42*(4), 335–345.

Marston, S. A. (2000). The social construction of scale. *Progress in Human Geography, 24*(2), 219–242.

Mayes, C. (2023). Healthy eating policy: Racial liberalism, global connections and contested science. *Food Ethics, 8*(1), 1.

Maysels, R., Figueroa Casas, A., Otero Sarmiento, J. D., & Zuñiga Meneses, S. M. (2023). Conceptualization of alternative food networks in Latin America: A case study of a local food system in Southwestern Colombia. *Frontiers in Sustainable Food Systems, 7*, 1216116.

McCutcheon, P. (2013). “Returning home to our rightful place”: The Nation of Islam and Muhammad Farms. *Geoforum, 49*, 61–70.

McCutcheon, P. (2019). Fannie Lou Hamer’s freedom farms and Black agrarian geographies. *Antipode, 51*(1), 207–224.

McCutcheon, P., Best, L. E., & Rajack-Talley, T. A. (Eds.). (2023). *Beyond the kitchen table: Black women and global food systems.* UNC Press Books.

McDaniel, E. (2009). *Politics in the pews: The political mobilization of Black churches.* University of Michigan Press.

McDonnell, S. (2020). Other dark sides of resilience: Politics and power in community-based efforts to strengthen resilience. *Anthropological Forum, 30*(1–2), 55–72.

McFetridge, S. (2022). Black farmers sue government for promised federal aid. *PBS News Hour.* https://www.pbs.org/newshour/politics/blackfarmers-sue-government-for-promised-federal-aid#:~:text=DES%20MOINES%2C%20Iowa%20(AP),to%20a%20class%2Daction% 20lawsuit

McGregor, J., & Rosenberg, E. (2020). Trump’s crackdown on training about white privilege draws broad opposition. *The Washington Post.* https://www.washingtonpost.com/business/2020/10/29/trump-diversity-training-labor-department/

McIntosh, W. A. (1996). *Sociologies of food and nutrition.* Springer Science & Business Media.

McKittrick, K. (2013). Plantation futures. *Small Axe: A Caribbean Journal of Criticism, 17* (42), 1–15.

Messer, C. M., Shriver, T. E., & Adams, A. E. (2018). The destruction of Black wall street: Tulsa’s 1921 riot and the eradication of accumulated wealth. *American Journal of Economics and Sociology, 77*(3–4), 789–819.

Millar, G. (2018). Decentring the intervention experts: Ethnographic peace research and policy engagement. *Cooperation and Conflict, 53*(2), 259–276.

Mishra, S. K., Khanal, A. R., & Collins, W. J. (2022). Farm-to-school programmes, benefits, health outcomes and barriers: A structured literature review. *Health Education Journal, 81*(7), 781–792.

Mol, A., & Law, J. (2007). Embodied action, enacted bodies: The example of hypoglycaemia. In R. V. Burri & J. Dumit (Eds.), *Biomedicine as culture: Instrumental practices, technoscientific knowledge, and new modes of life* (pp. 95–116). Routledge.

Möller, C. (2021). *Food charity and the psychologisation of poverty: Foucault in the food bank.* Routledge.

Morales, D. X., Morales, S. A., & Beltran, T. F. (2020). Racial/ethnic disparities in household food insecurity during the COVID-19 pandemic: A nationally representative study. *Journal of Racial and Ethnic Health Disparities, 8*(5), 1300–1314.

Morgan, W. T. W. (1963). The “white highlands” of Kenya. *The Geographical Journal, 129*(2), 140–155.

Moss, A. (2023). "Marching to save our children": Tammy Gray-Steele goes to Washington. *KFOR*. https://kfor.com/news/marching-to-save-our-children-tammy-gray-steele-goes-to-washington/

Mudege, N. N., Mdege, N., Abidin, P. E., & Bhatasara, S. (2017). The role of gender norms in access to agricultural training in Chikwawa and Phalombe, Malawi. *Gender, Place & Culture*, *24*(12), 1689–1710.

Muhammad, M., Wallerstein, N., Sussman, A. L., Avila, M., Belone, L., & Duran, B. (2015). Reflections on researcher identity and power: The impact of positionality on community based participatory research (CBPR) processes and outcomes. *Critical Sociology*, *41*(7–8), 1045–1063.

Mushquash, A. R., Pearson, E. S., Waddington, K., MacIsaac, A., Mohammed, S., Grassia, E., and Wekerle, C. (2021). User perspectives on a resilience-building app (JoyPop): Qualitative study. *JMIR mHealth and uHealth*, *9*(7), e28677.

Neff, R. A., Palmer, A. M., McKenzie, S. E., & Lawrence, R. S. (2009). Food systems and public health disparities. *Journal of Hunger & Environmental Nutrition*, *4*(3–4), 282–314.

Nesheim, M. C., Oria, M., & Yih, P. T. (Eds.). (2015). Overview of the U.S. food system (Chapter 2) In *A framework for assessing effects of the food system*. National Academies Press (US).

Norris, F. H., Stevens, S. P., Pfefferbaum, B., Wyche, K. F., & Pfefferbaum, R. L. (2008). Community resilience as a metaphor, theory, set of capacities, and strategy for disaster readiness. *American Journal of Community Psychology*, *41*, 127–150.

O'Grady Walshe, C. (2019). *Globalisation and seed sovereignty in Sub-Saharan Africa*. Springer.

O'Hara, S., & Toussaint, E. C. (2021). Food access in crisis: Food security and COVID-19. *Ecological Economics*, *180*, 106859.

Odoms-Young, A., & Bruce, M. A. (2018). Examining the impact of structural racism on food insecurity: Implications for addressing racial/ethnic disparities. *Family & Community Health*, *41*, S3–S6.

Olsen, O. H. (1962). The Ku Klux Klan: A study in reconstruction politics and propaganda. *The North Carolina Historical Review*, *39*(3), 340–362.

Orthel, B. D. (2022). Linking public health and heritage work. *International Journal of Heritage Studies*, *28*(1), 44–58.

Ottemöller, F. G., Matenga, T. F. L., Corbin, J. H., Nakhuda, H., Delobelle, P., Ayele, C., ... & Mweemba, O. (2021). Re-envisioning health promotion: Thinking and acting salutogenically towards equity for historically resilient communities. *Global Health Promotion*, *28*(4), 88–96.

Overend, A. (2020). *Shifting food facts: Dietary discourse in a post-truth culture*. Routledge.

Packalen, M., & Bhattacharya, J. (2020). NIH funding and the pursuit of edge science. *Proceedings of the National Academy of Sciences, 117*(22), 12011–12016.

Palmer, D., & Caldas, B. (2010). Critical ethnography. In K. King, Y.-J. Lai, & S. May (Eds.), *Research methods in language and education* (Encyclopedia of Language and Education, Vol. *10*, pp. 1–12).

Park, Y., Crath, R., & Jeffery, D. (2020). Disciplining the risky subject: A discourse analysis of the concept of resilience in social work literature. *Journal of Social Work, 20*(2), 152–172.

Parker, J., & Rathbone, R. (2007). *African history: A very short introduction* (Vol. 160). Oxford University Press.

Passidomo, C. (2013). Going "beyond food": Confronting structures of injustice in food systems research and praxis. *Journal of Agriculture, Food Systems, and Community Development, 3*(4), 89–93.

Peck, J., & Tickell, A. (2002). Neoliberalizing space. *Antipode, 34*(3), 380–404.

Penniman, L. (2018). *Farming while black: Soul fire farm's practical guide to liberation on the land.* Chelsea Green Publishing.

Penniman, L. (2022). Black land matters. *Transition, 133*, 20–32.

Perry, K. K., & Sealey-Huggins, L. (2023). Racial capitalism and climate justice: White redemptive power and the uneven geographies of eco-imperial crisis. *Geoforum, 145*, 103772.

Pettinger, C., Hunt, L., Gardiner, H., Garg, P., Howard, L., & Wagstaff, C. (2024). Engaging with "less affluent"communities for food system transformation: A community food researcher model (FoodSEqual project). *Proceedings of the Nutrition Society, 83*(3), 180–194.

Pfeffer, F. T., & Killewald, A. (2018). Generations of advantage. Multigenerational correlations in family wealth. *Social Forces, 96*(4), 1411–1442.

Pfefferbaum, R. L., Pfefferbaum, B., Van Horn, R. L., Klomp, R. W., Norris, F. H., & Reissman, D. B. (2013). The communities advancing resilience toolkit (CART): An intervention to build community resilience to disasters. *Journal of Public Health Management and Practice, 19*(3), 250–258.

Putnam, R. D. (2000). Bowling alone: America's declining social capital. In L. Crothers & C. Lockhart (Eds.), *Culture and politics: A reader* (pp. 223–234). Palgrave Macmillan.

Quaicoe, O., Asiseh, F., Baffoe-Bonnie, A., & Ng'ombe, J. N. (2024). Small farms in North Carolina, United States: Analyzing farm and operator characteristics in the pursuit of economic resilience and sustainability. *Applied Economic Perspectives and Policy, 46*(1), 13–31.

Quinn, K. G., Dickson-Gomez, J., Pearson, B., Marion, E., Amikrhanian, Y., & Kelly, J. A. (2022). Intersectional resilience among Black gay, bisexual, and other men who have sex with men, Wisconsin and Ohio, 2019. *American Journal of Public Health, 112*(S4), S405–S412.

Ramírez, M. M. (2015). The elusive inclusive: Black food geographies and racialized food spaces. *Antipode, 47*(3), 748–769.

Rampersad, G., Goodall, K., Simmons, T., & Kinderknecht, K. (2022). *Prioritizing health equity & food security*. Feeding America.

Ranganathan, M., & Bratman, E. (2021). From urban resilience to abolitionist climate justice in Washington, DC. *Antipode, 53*(1), 115–137.

Ranta, R., Colás, A., & Monterescu, D. (Eds.). (2022). *"Going native?": Settler colonialism and food*. Palgrave Macmillan.

Raschke, V., & Cheema, B. (2008). Colonisation, the New World Order, and the eradication of traditional food habits in East Africa: Historical perspective on the nutrition transition. *Public Health Nutrition, 11*(7), 662–674.

Rasmussen, C. A. (2024). "How many Black hippies do you see?" The counterculture in black and white. *Journal of American Studies, 58*(2), 275–300.

Reese, A. M., & Cooper, D. (2021). Making spaces something like freedom: Black feminist praxis in the re/imagining of a just food system. *ACME: An International Journal for Critical Geographies, 20*(4), 450–459.

Reid, D. A. (2007). *Reaping a greater harvest: African Americans, the extension service, and rural reform in Jim Crow Texas* (Vol. 14). Texas A&M University Press.

Reid, D. A., & Bennett, E. P. (Eds.). (2012). *Beyond forty acres and a mule: African American landowning families since reconstruction*. University Press of Florida.

Reiley, L. (2021). Relief bill is most significant legislation for Black farmers since Civil Rights Act, experts say. *The Washington Post*. https://www.washingtonpost.com/business/2021/03/08/reparations-black-farmers-stimulus/

Reynolds, B. J. (2002). *Black farmers in America, 1865-2000: The pursuit of independent farming and the role of cooperatives* (Vol. 194). US Department of Agriculture, Rural Business-Cooperative Service.

Rice, A. M., Einbinder, N., & Calderón, C. I. (2023). "With agroecology, we can defend ourselves": Examining campesino resilience and economic solidarity during pandemic-era economic shock in Guatemala. *Agroecology and Sustainable Food Systems, 47*(2), 273–305.

Riddle, W. A. (1995). The origins of black sharecropping. *The Mississippi Quarterly, 49*(1), 53–71.

Riley, W. J. (2012). Health disparities: Gaps in access, quality and affordability of medical care. *Transactions of the American Clinical and Climatological Association, 123*, 167.

Roberts, A. E. (2021). Who belongs in Indian Territory? *The Journal of the Gilded Age and Progressive Era, 20*(2), 334–337.

Robins, J. (2016). *Cotton and race across the Atlantic: Britain, Africa, and America, 1900-1920* (Vol. 73). Boydell & Brewer.

Roessler, P., Pengl, Y., Marty, R., Titlow, K., & Van de Walle, N. (2020). *The cash crop revolution, colonialism and legacies of spatial inequality: Evidence from Africa.* Centre for the Study of African Economies.

Roessler, P., Pengl, Y. I., Marty, R., Titlow, K. S., & van de Walle, N. (2022). The cash crop revolution, colonialism and economic reorganization in Africa. *World Development, 158*, 105934.

Rotz, S., Duncan, E., Small, M., Botschner, J., Dara, R., Mosby, I., and Fraser, E. D. (2019). The politics of digital agricultural technologies: A preliminary review. *Sociologia Ruralis, 59*(2), 203–229.

Sarauw, J. (2024). Op-Ed: State of the Territory | The fight for land and identity in the U.S. Virgin Islands: Gentrification in the wake of natural disasters. *The St. Thomas Source.* https://stthomassource.com/content/2024/10/27/op-ed-state-of-the-territory-the-fight-for-land-and-identity-in-the-u-s-virgin-islands-gentrification-in-the-wake-of-natural-disasters/

Sastry, S., Stephenson, M., Dillon, P., & Carter, A. (2021). A meta-theoretical systematic review of the culture-centered approach to health communication: Toward a refined, "nested" model. *Communication Theory, 31*(3), 380–421.

Scordato, L., & Gulbrandsen, M. (2024). Resilience perspectives in sustainability transitions research: A systematic literature review. *Environmental Innovation and Societal Transitions, 52*, 100887.

Scott, W. R. (1995). *Institutions and organizations: Ideas, interests, and identities.* Sage Publications.

Scott, L. O. (2009). Challenging the American conscience, re-imagining American identity. In D. Field (Ed.), *A Historical Guide to James Baldwin* (pp. 141–176). Oxford University Press.

Seguin, R. A., Morgan, E. H., Hanson, K. L., Ammerman, A. S., Jilcott Pitts, S. B., Kolodinsky, J., ... & McGuirt, J. T. (2017). Farm Fresh Foods for Healthy Kids (F3HK): An innovative community supported agriculture intervention to prevent childhood obesity in low-income families and strengthen local agricultural economies. *BMC Public Health, 17*, 1–20.

Sharma, V., & Sharma, R. (2024). Food is medicine initiative for mitigating food insecurity in the United States. *Journal of Preventive Medicine and Public Health, 57*(2), 96.

Shaw, J., McLean, K. C., Taylor, B., Swartout, K., & Querna, K. (2016). Beyond resilience: Why we need to look at systems too. *Psychology of Violence, 6*(1), 34.

Shiva, V. (2001). *Stolen harvest: The hijacking of the global food supply.* Zed Books.

Sinclair, W. (1984). Laxity, confusion mar USDA rights program. *Washington Post*. https://www.washingtonpost.com/archive/politics/1984/07/10/laxity-confusion-mar-usda-rights-program/dc532022-dc89-4fa4-863e-3361cb9bd8a5/

Slavchevska, V., Doss, C. R., de la O Campos A. P, and Brunelli, C. (2021). Beyond ownership: Women's and men's land rights in Sub-Saharan Africa. *Oxford Development Studies*, *49*(1), 2–22.

Slocum, R. (2007). Whiteness, space and alternative food practice. *Geoforum*, *38*(3), 520–533.

Small, Z. (2020). Through art, I hope that we can make one Tulsa. *New York Times*. https://www.nytimes.com/2020/06/26/arts/design/tulsa-greenwood-artists.html

Smith, B. J. (2019). Building emancipatory food power: Freedom farms, rocky acres, and the struggle for food justice. *Journal of Agriculture, Food Systems, and Community Development*, *8*(4), 33–43.

Smith, R. A. J., & Rhiney, K. (2016). Climate (in) justice, vulnerability and livelihoods in the Caribbean: The case of the indigenous Caribs in northeastern St. Vincent. *Geoforum*, *73*, 22–31.

Smolski, A. R., & Schulman, M. D. (2024). Navigating farm stress: Traumatic and resilient dimensions of the Black agrarian frame. *Journal of Agromedicine*, *29*(1), 55–65.

Sousa, E. C., & Raizada, M. N. (2020). Contributions of African crops to American culture and beyond: The slave trade and other journeys of resilient peoples and crops. *Frontiers in Sustainable Food Systems*, *4*, 586340.

Stokols, D., Lejano, R. P., & Hipp, J. (2013). Enhancing the resilience of human–environment systems: A social ecological perspective. *Ecology and Society*, *18*(1), 7–22.

Stolberg, S. G. (2025). Group of experts says RFK Jr. would "significantly undermine" public health. *New York Times*. https://www.nytimes.com/2025/01/13/us/politics/robert-f-kennedy-jr-public-health-secretary.html

Suchman, M. C. (1995). Managing legitimacy: Strategic and institutional approaches. *Academy of Management Review*, *20*(3), 571–610.

Sumberg, J., & Giller, K. E. (2022). What is "conventional"agriculture? *Global Food Security*, *32*, 100617.

Suslovic, B., & Lett, E. (2024). Resilience is an adverse event: A critical discussion of resilience theory in health services research and public health. *Community Health Equity Research & Policy*, *44*(3), 339–343.

Taylor, S. C., Smernoff, Z. L., Rajan, M., Steeman, S., Gehringer, B. N., Dow, H. C., ... & Brodkin, E. S. (2022). Investigating the relationships between resilience, autism-related quantitative traits, and mental health outcomes among adults during the COVID-19 pandemic. *Journal of Psychiatric Research*, *148*, 250–257.

Terui, S., Divya, S., & Acheampong, B. F. (2023). Language-discordance as a barrier to health equity. In B. J. Van Gilder, J. T. Austin & J. S. Bruscella (Eds.), *Communication and organizational changemaking for diversity, equity, and inclusion: A case studies approach* (pp. 61–77). Routledge.

Theodoridis, D., Rönnbäck, K., & Galli, S. (2024). The failed promise of freedom—Emancipation and wealth inequality in the Caribbean. *The Economic History Review*, *78*(3), 952–974.

Thompson, P. O., Omitayo, A., Ademu, L. O., & Maiangwa, B. (2024). African folklore: A tool for improving sustainable resource management practices in Africa. *Environmental Development*, *51*, 101044.

Thurland, K. C. (2014). *The sugar industry on St. Croix*. Author House.

Tomich, D. W. (Ed.). (2016). *The politics of the second slavery*. SUNY Press.

Tornaghi, C., & Dehaene, M. (2020). The prefigurative power of urban political agroecology: Rethinking the urbanisms of agroecological transitions for food system transformation. *Agroecology and Sustainable Food Systems*, *44*(5), 594–610.

Tseng, T. W. J., Robinson, B. E., Bellemare, M. F., BenYishay, A., Blackman, A., Boucher, T., ... & Masuda, Y. J. (2021). Influence of land tenure interventions on human well-being and environmental outcomes. *Nature Sustainability*, *4*(3), 242–251.

Tsige, M., Synnevåg, G., & Aune, J. B. (2020). Gendered constraints for adopting climate-smart agriculture amongst smallholder Ethiopian women farmers. *Scientific African*, *7*, e00250.

Tyler, S. (2020). Rematriating to the wombs of the world. In C. E. Sachs, L. Jensen, P. Castellanos, & K. Sexsmith (Eds.), *Routledge handbook of gender and agriculture* (pp. 410–418). Routledge.

Tyler, S., & Fraser, A. (2016). Womanism and agroecology: An intersectional praxis seed keeping as acts of political warfare. In P. Godfrey, and D. Torres (Eds.), *Emergent possibilities for global sustainability* (pp. 19–30). Routledge.

Tyler, S. S., & Moore, E. A. (2013). Plight of Black farmers in the context of USDA farm loan programs: A research agenda for the future. *Professional Agricultural Workers Journal*, *1*(1), 6.

Ugwu, P. (2019). Women in agriculture: Challenges facing women in African farming. In *Project report of African women in agriculture*. https://www.researchgate.net/publication/332053861_women_in_agriculture_challenges_facing_women_in_african_farming.

United States Department of Agriculture (2025). *Secretary Rollins Takes Bold Action to Stop Wasteful Spending and Optimize USDA to Better Serve American Agriculture*. https://www.usda.gov/about-usda/news/press-releases/2025/02/14/secretary-rollins-takes-bold-action-stop-wasteful-spending-and-optimize-usda-better-serve-american

United States Department of Agriculture (n.d.), Urban agriculture. *Natural Agriculture Library*. https://www.nal.usda.gov/farms-and-agricultural-production-systems/urban-agriculture

United States Department of Agriculture Natural Agricultural Statistics Service (2017a). *Black producers*. US Department of Agriculture, National Agricultural Statistics Service.

United States Department of Agriculture Natural Agricultural Statistics Service (2017b). *Female producers*. US Department of Agriculture, National Agricultural Statistics Service.

United States Government Accountability Office (2008). *U.S. Department of Agriculture: Management of civil rights efforts continues to be deficient despite years of attention*. https://www.gao.gov/assets/a120067.html

United States Government Accountability Office (2013). *Congressionally chartered organizations: Key principles for leveraging nonfederal resources*. https://www.gao.gov/products/gao-13-549

Vecco, M. (2010). A definition of cultural heritage: From the tangible to the intangible. *Journal of Cultural Heritage*, *11*(3), 321–324.

Volcovici, V., Lynch, S., & Mason, J. (2025). Trump administration cuts environmental justice programs at EPA, DOJ. *Reuters*. https://www.reuters.com/world/us/trump-administration-cuts-environmental-justice-programs-epa-doj-sources-say-2025-02-06/

Waites, B. (2005). *Europe and the wider world*. Routledge.

Wallance, G. (2021). Racial reparations at the USDA. *The Hill*. https://thehill.com/opinion/civil-rights/559586-racial-reparations-at-the-usda/

Wamble, J. J. (2025). *We choose you: How Black voters decide which candidates to support*. Cambridge University Press.

Wells-Barnett, I. B. (1894). *The red record: Tabulated statistics and alleged causes of lynchings in the United States, 1892–1893–1894*. Donohue & Henneberry. Retrieved November 23, 2020, from Frederick Douglass Papers, Library of Congress, Manuscript Division.

White, M. M. (2011). Environmental reviews & case studies: D-town farm: African American resistance to food insecurity and the transformation of Detroit. *Environmental Practice*, *13*(4), 406–417.

White, I. K., & Laird, C. N. (2020). *Steadfast democrats: How social forces shape Black political behavior*. Princeton University Press.

Whitehouse.gov (2023). FACT SHEET: The Biden-Harris administration advances equity and opportunity for Black Americans and communities across the country. https://www.whitehouse.gov/briefing-room/statements-releases/2023/02/27/fact-sheet-the-biden-%E2%81%A0harris-administration-advances-equity-and-opportunity-for-black-americans-and-communities-across-the-country/

Whitehouse.gov (2025). EXECUTIVE ORDER: Ending radical and wasteful government DEI programs and preferencing. https://www.whitehouse.gov/presidential-actions/2025/01/ending-radical-and-wasteful-government-dei-programs-and-preferencing/

Widgren, M. (2017). Agricultural intensification in Sub-Saharan Africa, 1500–1800. In G. Austin (Ed.), *Economic development and environmental history in the Anthropocene: Perspectives on Asia and Africa* (pp. 51–67). Bloomsbury Academic.

Wile, R. (2024). WNBA players could earn more money, but it will take big changes to make that happen: Despite its momentum, the WNBA still generates only a small fraction of the revenue the NBA does, making it tough for women's pay to reach parity with men's. *NBC News*. https://www.nbcnews.com/business/business-news/women-basketball-players-pay-discrepancy-record-viewership-explained-rcna148233

Williams, A. L. (2022). The heritage strikes back: Athlete activism, Black Lives Matter, and the iconic fifth wave of activism in the (W) NBA bubble. *Cultural Studies↔ Critical Methodologies*, *22*(3), 266–275.

Williams, J. (2021). *Climate change is racist: Race, privilege and the struggle for climate justice*. Icon Books.

Williams, J. M., & Holt-Giménez, E. (Eds.). (2017). *Land justice: Re-imagining land, food, and the commons*. Food First Books.

Wise, T. A. (2020). *Failing Africa's farmers: An impact assessment of the Alliance for a Green Revolution in Africa.* (Global Development and Environment Institute Working Paper No. 20-01). Tufts University. https://bpb-us-e1.wpmucdn.com/sites.tufts.edu/dist/0/5123/files/2020/07/20-01_Wise_FailureToYield.pdf

Wood, S. D., & Gilbert, J. (2000). Returning African American farmers to the land: Recent trends and a policy rationale. *The Review of Black Political Economy*, *27*(4), 43–64.

Wood, S. D., & Ragar, C. R. (2012). Grass tops democracy: Institutional discrimination in the civil rights violations of Black farmers. *Journal of Pan African Studies*, *5*(6), 16–36.

Woods-Jaeger, B., Siedlik, E., Adams, A., Piper, K., O'Connor, P., & Berkley-Patton, J. (2020). Building a contextually-relevant understanding of resilience among African American youth exposed to community violence. *Behavioral Medicine*, *46*(3–4), 330–339.

World Bank (2022). The fight against food insecurity in the Caribbean. https://www.worldbank.org/en/news/feature/2022/06/28/food-insecurity-caribbean

World Food Programme (2023). Cash transfers. https://www.wfp.org/cash-transfers

Wright, K. E., Lucero, J. E., Ferguson, J. K., Granner, M. L., Devereux, P. G., Pearson, J. L., & Crosbie, E. (2021). The impact that cultural food security has on identity and well-being in the second-generation US American minority college students. *Food Security*, *13*, 701–715.

Wudil, A. H., Usman, M., Rosak-Szyrocka, J., Pilař, L., & Boye, M. (2022). Reversing years for global food security: a review of the food security situation in Sub-Saharan Africa (SSA). *International Journal of Environmental Research and Public Health*, *19*(22), 14836.

Young, I. M. (1990). *Justice and the politics of difference*. Princeton University Press.

Zavala, A. (2024). "A complete betrayal": CA reparations task force leader responds to Legislative Black Caucus decision to block bills. *KCRA*. https://www.kcra.com/article/ca-reparations-task-force-leader-responds-black-caucus-block-bills/62049034

Zhang, R., & Mei, X. (2024). Neo-green imperialism: The development of Virgin Islands National Park. *Environmental History*, *29*(4), 701–724.

Zimmerman, M. A., & Zeitz, G. J. (2002). Beyond survival: Achieving new venture growth by building legitimacy. *Academy of Management Review*, *27*(3), 414–431.